Single Best Answer Questions for Dentistry

Single Best Answer Questions for Dentistry

(Formerly *MCQs in Dentistry*)

Over 280 single best answer questions across nine key dental subject areas

Prateek Biyani, BDS (Hons.), MFDS RCPS(Glasg.), Cert Med Ed

Specialty Doctor (Oral and Maxillofacial Surgery);
Associate Dentist
Chesterfield Royal Hospital
Chesterfield/Sheffield, UK

WILEY Blackwell

Registered Office
John Wiley & Sons, Inc., 111 River Street, Hoboken, NJ 07030, USA
John Wiley & Sons Ltd, The Atrium, Southern Gate, Chichester, West Sussex, PO19 8SQ, UK

Editorial Office
9600 Garsington Road, Oxford, OX4 2DQ, UK

For details of our global editorial offices, customer services, and more information about Wiley products visit us at www.wiley.com.

Wiley also publishes its books in a variety of electronic formats and by print-on-demand. Some content that appears in standard print versions of this book may not be available in other formats.

Library of Congress Cataloging-in-Publication Data

Names: Biyani, Prateek, author.
Title: Single best answer questions for dentistry / Prateek Biyani.
Description: Hoboken, NJ : Wiley-Blackwell, 2020. | Includes index.
Identifiers: LCCN 2020023348 (print) | LCCN 2020023349 (ebook) | ISBN 9781119702351 (paperback) | ISBN 9781119702344 (adobe pdf) | ISBN 9781119702375 (epub)
Subjects: MESH: Dentistry | Examination Questions
Classification: LCC RK57 (print) | LCC RK57 (ebook) | NLM WU 18.2 | DDC 617.60076–dc23
LC record available at https://lccn.loc.gov/2020023348
LC ebook record available at https://lccn.loc.gov/2020023349

Cover Design: Wiley
Cover Images: Dental Check-up © Branimir76/Getty Images, Dentist medical tools on tray © baona/Getty Images

Set in 9/11.5pt Meridien by SPi Global, Pondicherry, India
Printed and bound in Singapore by Markono Print Media Pte Ltd

10 9 8 7 6 5 4 3 2 1

Contents

Preface

Practising questions is an important aspect of revision. This book aims to provide a useful source of revision for dental students and those sitting the MJDF/MFDS/ORE exams. It features questions with the corresponding answers on the next page. Knowledge in this book is accurate at the time of writing and at the level of that which would be required for the current examinations but, as would be expected, this content may be updated over the years.

Mr Prateek Biyani
BDS (Hons.), MFDS RCPS(Glasg.), Cert Med Ed

CHAPTER 1

Restorative Dentistry

1. What is the ideal freeway space (FWS) for complete dentures?
   (a) 1–3 mm
   (b) 2–4 mm
   (c) 3–5 mm
   (d) 4–6 mm
   (e) 5–7 mm

2. Which of the following describes a Kennedy Class II, in Kennedy's classification for partially dentate patients?
   (a) Patient with bilateral free-end saddles
   (b) Patient with a unilateral free-end saddle
   (c) Patient with a unilateral bounded saddle
   (d) Patient with an anterior bounded saddle
   (e) Patient with a bilateral free-end saddle and a missing UR2

3. What is the primary purpose of indirect retention in partial denture design?
   (a) Prevent displacement of the denture in the axial direction
   (b) Aid insertion and removal of the denture
   (c) Prevent lateral forces on teeth
   (d) Prevent tipping/rotation of the denture about a fulcrum
   (e) Allow for effective cleaning

4. A sclerosed canal can be more easily navigated using which of the following irrigants?
   (a) Chlorhexidine
   (b) Sodium hypochlorite
   (c) Ethylenediaminetetraacetic acid (EDTA)
   (d) Water
   (e) Calcium hydroxide

5. Which graph best describes the changes in plaque pH in response to food?
   (a) The Miller Curve
   (b) The Monson Curve
   (c) The Stephan Curve
   (d) The David Curve
   (e) The Spee Curve

1. b

This is the ideal FWS. However, often, if patients have had a different FWS for a long period of time, it may be necessary to adhere to their existing FWS. This is primarily to ensure good habituation.

2. b

Kennedy Class II is a unilateral free-end saddle. It may also have modifications. It is only Kennedy Class IV that does not have any modifications, as the most posterior saddle dictates the class and, thus, any modifications would in fact fall in to a different class.

3. d

Indirect retention helps prevent tipping of the denture about a fulcrum created by the denture components. It can be provided by other denture components including clasps, rests and connectors.

4. c

EDTA is a chelating agent used to soften the dentine and allow easy exploration of sclerosed canals. Sodium hypochlorite is the typical irrigant for root canal treatments. Calcium hydroxide is better used in a pulpless, temporary dressing.

5. c

The curve demonstrating plaque pH changes associated with snacking is the Stephan Curve. This helps demonstrate how frequent snacking causes the pH to drop below the critical pH more frequently. As a result, an individual is more likely to develop caries.

6. Which of the following is the advancing edge of a carious lesion in enamel?
   (a) Dark zone
   (b) Body of the lesion
   (c) Surface zone
   (d) Translucent zone
   (e) Zone of sclerosis

7. Which of the following is a crucial feature of amalgam cavity design?
   (a) 110° cavo-surface angle
   (b) Presence of unsupported enamel
   (c) Leaving caries at the amelo-dentinal junction (ADJ)
   (d) Placement of pins
   (e) Undercuts

8. Which of the following best describes retruded contact position (RCP)?
   (a) The position of the mandible, relative to the maxilla, when the teeth are maximally intercuspated
   (b) The first tooth contact when the condyle lies in its most favourable position in the glenoid fossa
   (c) The position of the mandible when the condyle lies in its most favourable position in the glenoid fossa
   (d) The movement of the mandible during protrusive movements
   (e) The movement of the mandible during lateral movements

9. Which of the following is not a feature of the ideal occlusion?
   (a) Mutual protection
   (b) Molar guidance
   (c) Anterior guidance
   (d) RCP = ICP
   (e) Forces down the long axis of the teeth

10. A patient presents with pain brought on by hot/cold stimuli that settles shortly after the stimulus is removed. What is the likely diagnosis?
    (a) Reversible pulpitis
    (b) Acute irreversible pulpitis
    (c) Chronic irreversible pulpitis
    (d) Periapical abscess
    (e) Cracked tooth syndrome

6. d

The translucent zone marks the advancing edge of a carious lesion in enamel. This is then followed by the dark zone, the body of the lesion and finally the surface zone.

7. e

Undercuts are necessary for amalgam restorations as they rely on mechanical retention. A 90° cavo-surface angle is needed to reduce the risk of fracture, due to thin amalgam sections, and caries should always be cleared from the ADJ.

8. b

RCP is the position where first tooth contact occurs with the mandible in centric relation, i.e. where the mandibular condyle lies in the most superior (comfortable) position in the glenoid fossa.

9. b

An ideal occlusion should feature canine guidance, and not molar guidance, for lateral excursions. This protects the posterior teeth.

10. a

This is a classic symptom of reversible pulpitis – pain settling once the stimulus is removed. The causative factor, for example a leaking restoration, needs to be corrected for symptoms to settle.

11. Which of the following is not a method of determining working length?
   (a) Apex locator
   (b) Paper points
   (c) Preoperative radiograph
   (d) Working length radiograph
   (e) Step-back technique

12. Which of the following irrigants helps remove the smear layer during root canal treatment?
   (a) Sodium hypochlorite
   (b) Water
   (c) Chlorhexidine
   (d) EDTA
   (e) Saline

13. Which of the following is not a contraindication for surgical endodontics?
   (a) Persistent disease where non-surgical treatments have failed
   (b) Poor surgical access
   (c) Unrestorable tooth
   (d) Underlying bleeding disorders
   (e) Non-surgical treatments are feasible

14. Which of the following is unlikely to cause insecurity of a complete denture?
   (a) Overextension in the buccal sulcus
   (b) Lack of denture extension
   (c) Balanced occlusion and articulation
   (d) Extension over the hamular notch
   (e) Thin post-dam

15. Which of the following is a contraindication for veneers?
   (a) Diastema closure
   (b) Fluorosis
   (c) Camouflaging a canine as a lateral incisor
   (d) Pulpless teeth
   (e) Good oral hygiene

11. e

Step-back technique is a method of root canal preparation and not a method of determining working length.

12. d

EDTA helps remove the smear layer which allows irrigants in to the dentinal tubules. This allows more thorough chemo-mechanical preparation.

13. a

Persistent disease, where standard treatment has failed, is the general reason for carrying out surgical endodontics. All the other options are common contraindications.

14. c

Balanced occlusion and articulation are the desired occlusal schemes with dentures and lead to best stability. All the other options are likely to lead to a lack of retention in some form.

15. d

Pulpless teeth will generally continue to discolour over time and so the aesthetic value of a veneer will be lost. Careful consideration must be given to these teeth.

16. Which of the following would be an indication for crown placement?
   (a) More conservative options available
   (b) Subgingival caries
   (c) Grade 2 mobility
   (d) Heavily restored tooth
   (e) Root fracture

17. What is the ideal degree of taper for preparation of an indirect restoration?
   (a) 1–3°
   (b) 3–5°
   (c) 5–7°
   (d) 7–9°
   (e) >9°

18. Erosion means loss of tooth surface tissue due to:
   (a) Chemical processes independent of bacteria
   (b) Chemical processes associated with bacteria
   (c) Tooth-to-tooth contact
   (d) Damage from foreign bodies
   (e) Occlusal forces

19. Which of the following is an indication for the use of rubber dam?
   (a) Latex allergy
   (b) Claustrophobia
   (c) Difficult access
   (d) Airway protection
   (e) Improving impression detail

20. What is the usual shoulder preparation for a metal-ceramic crown?
   (a) 0.5 mm
   (b) 1.0 mm
   (c) 1.3 mm
   (d) 1.8 mm
   (e) 2.0 mm

16. d

A heavily restored tooth, without any recurrent caries, would be an ideal candidate for a crown. If there is a more conservative management option then this should be attempted first. Extensive caries and periodontal disease are strict contraindications.

17. c

A taper of 5–7° is ideal to allow for optimal retention.

18. a

Erosion occurs due to chemical processes independent of bacteria. Attrition is due to tooth-to-tooth contact and abrasion is due to foreign bodies (very commonly toothbrushing trauma).

19. d

Airway protection is critical in root canal preparation. Other indications include moisture isolation and improved visibility.

20. c

A general shoulder preparation of between 1.2–1.5 mm should be done to ensure adequate thickness and space for metal and porcelain.

21. Which of the following is not a principle of crown preparation?
    (a) Undercut preparation
    (b) Conservative preparation
    (c) Retention form
    (d) Resistance form
    (e) Marginal integrity

22. What is the optimum crown-root ratio for crown preparation?
    (a) 1:1
    (b) 1:2
    (c) 2:3
    (d) 2:1
    (e) 3:2

23. Which of the following is not used as a temporary following indirect restoration preparation?
    (a) Amalgam
    (b) Direct composite
    (c) Stainless steel crown
    (d) Polycarbonate shell crown
    (e) Aluminium shell crown

24. What is the shortened dental arch (SDA)?
    (a) 4–5 pairs of occluding teeth
    (b) 6–7 pairs of occluding teeth
    (c) 7–8 pairs of occluding teeth
    (d) 9–10 pairs of occluding teeth
    (e) 11–12 pairs of occluding teeth

25. What is bracing in relation to partial dentures?
    (a) Resistance to lateral and anterior displacing forces
    (b) Resistance to axial displacing forces
    (c) Resistance to tipping of denture
    (d) Resistance to displacement of denture in to the ridge
    (e) Ability to connect denture components

21. a

Undercuts should be avoided for conventional crown preparations to ensure proper seating and retention.

22. c

Ideally there should be a ratio of 2 : 3 in order to have a more predictable outcome. However, 1 : 1 may be accepted but caution is advised.

23. a

Amalgam is never used as a temporary following indirect preparation, as it cannot be constructed in the appropriate shape.

24. d

The SDA typically refers to 9–10 pairs of occluding teeth, allowing adequate function for a patient. This may inform treatment planning for missing teeth.

25. a

Bracing prevents the denture from being displaced laterally and anteriorly. It can be provided by major connectors, clasps and reciprocating plates.

26. Which of the following is not an advantage of an overdenture compared to a complete denture?
(a) Improved proprioception
(b) Better aesthetics
(c) Increased support from roots
(d) Preservation of bone
(e) Increased retention via precision attachments

27. What is the minimum thickness needed for incisal and occlusal rest seats?
(a) 0.2 mm
(b) 0.5 mm
(c) 0.7 mm
(d) 1.0 mm
(e) 1.5 mm

28. Which bur can be used to widen endodontic access cavities without damaging the floor?
(a) Rosehead
(b) Gates-Glidden
(c) Microfine diamond
(d) Endo-Z
(e) Tungsten carbide

29. What is the fluoride content of fluoride varnish?
(a) 1200 ppm
(b) 2200 ppm
(c) 5600 ppm
(d) 10 200 ppm
(e) 22 600 ppm

30. What is the NICE recall interval for high caries risk patients?
(a) 1 month
(b) 3 months
(c) 12 months
(d) 24 months
(e) 36 months

26. b

There is not an aesthetic advantage of an overdenture over a complete denture.

27. b

A minimum of 0.5 mm is required to provide sufficient thickness of the rest, otherwise fracture is likely. This may require rest seats to be cut in the relevant teeth or assessment for sufficient occlusal space without preparation.

28. d

Endo-Z burs have a non-cutting tip which allows for access preparation without risk of perforating the floor.

29. e

Fluoride varnish can be applied up to four times a year on high-risk patients and contains 22 600 ppm of fluoride.

30. b

A three-month recall should be put in place for high caries risk patients until they are stabilised.

31. Which of the following is not a property of mineral trioxide aggregate (MTA)?
   (a) Non-toxic
   (b) Non-resorbable
   (c) Short setting time
   (d) Biocompatible
   (e) Minimal marginal leakage

32. Which of the following describes the obturation technique of warm vertical condensation?
   (a) Obturation with a single master gutta percha (GP) cone with sealer
   (b) Obturation with a master cone and GP accessory points, using an ultrasonic unit to warm the GP
   (c) Obturation using a reverse H-file to push GP down the canal
   (d) Obturation with a plastic carrier coated in GP
   (e) Obturation with a downpack/apical plug and then backfilling incrementally with melted GP

33. What is the average length of a maxillary canine?
   (a) 20.5 mm
   (b) 21.6 mm
   (c) 24.7 mm
   (d) 28.3 mm
   (e) 26.5 mm

34. What is the suggested concentration for chlorhexidine as a root canal irrigant?
   (a) 0.001%
   (b) 0.1–1%
   (c) 0.2–2%
   (d) 2–3%
   (e) 3.5–5%

31. c

MTA has a long setting time, which is one of its main disadvantages. Biodentine is an alternative material that aims to improve on this property primarily through the addition of calcium chloride.

32. e

Warm vertical condensation involves placing an apical plug for apical control and then backfilling from this. Option **a** describes single cone technique; **b** describes warm lateral condensation; **c** describes thermomechanical compaction; and **d** describes carrier-based systems.

33. e

The average length of a maxillary canine is 26.5 mm with, typically, a single root and single root canal. Mandibular canines are usually slightly shorter at 25.6 mm.

34. c

Chlorhexidine should be used at a concentration of 0.2–2%. Chlorhexidine 2% has the same antibacterial activity as 5.25% sodium hypochlorite, with residual effects lasting for up to 48 hours.

CHAPTER 2
Oral Medicine

Single Best Answer Questions for Dentistry, First Edition. Prateek Biyani.
© 2021 John Wiley & Sons Ltd. Published 2021 by John Wiley & Sons Ltd.

1. Which of the following is a common differential diagnosis of a pyogenic granuloma?
   (a) Peripheral giant cell granuloma
   (b) Fibrous polyp
   (c) Lipoma
   (d) Dental abscess
   (e) Squamous cell papilloma

2. Which of the following drugs is not associated with gingival hyperplasia?
   (a) Nifedipine
   (b) Phenytoin
   (c) Ciclosporin
   (d) Aspirin
   (e) Amlodipine

3. Which of the following is not a common cause of angular cheilitis?
   (a) Candidal infection
   (b) Hypothyroidism
   (c) Vitamin B12 deficiency
   (d) Folate deficiency
   (e) Iron deficiency

4. A 50-year-old man presents with multiple crusting lesions and ulcers on the left side of his face. He noticed a tingling sensation beforehand and the rash has been present for a week. Which virus is a potential cause?
   (a) Herpes simplex I
   (b) Herpes zoster
   (c) Cytomegalovirus
   (d) Coxsackie A
   (e) Epstein–Barr

5. Which virus is associated with development of hairy leukoplakia?
   (a) Human papillomavirus
   (b) Herpes simplex I
   (c) Hepatitis B
   (d) Epstein–Barr
   (e) Cytomegalovirus

1. a

Both are characterised as highly vascular lesions with very similar clinical presentations, typically presenting on the gingivae.

2. d

Aspirin has not been associated with gingival hyperplasia. All the other drugs are common causes.

3. b

Iron, B12 and folate deficiency are common causes of angular cheilitis. Often there is an associated candidal/*Staphylococcus aureus* infection.

4. b

This is most likely shingles caused by reactivation of the varicella zoster virus. It most often presents in older patients, along one or more divisions of the trigeminal nerve on the face. It generally stops at the midline and lasts 2–3 weeks.

5. d

Epstein–Barr is associated with development of hairy leukoplakia, which usually presents in HIV/AIDS patients. It is also associated with infectious mononucleosis, Burkitt's lymphoma and nasopharyngeal carcinoma.

6. What type of lesion would acute pseudomembranous candidiasis present as?
   (a) Erythematous patches
   (b) Circular ulcers
   (c) White plaques that can be removed
   (d) White plaques that cannot be removed
   (e) Vesicular lesions

7. Which form of candidal infection has a risk of becoming malignant?
   (a) Acute pseudomembranous candidiasis
   (b) Acute atrophic candidiasis
   (c) Chronic atrophic candidiasis
   (d) Chronic hyperplastic candidiasis
   (e) Median rhomboid glossitis

8. Pemphigus is an example of which type of hypersensitivity?
   (a) Type I hypersensitivity
   (b) Type II hypersensitivity
   (c) Type III hypersensitivity
   (d) Type IV hypersensitivity
   (e) Type V hypersensitivity

9. Target lesions are commonly seen in which of the following conditions?
   (a) Pemphigus
   (b) Pemphigoid
   (c) Lichen planus
   (d) Erythema multiforme
   (e) Lichenoid reactions

10. Which of the following features is not common in minor recurrent aphthous stomatitis (RAS)?
    (a) Occurs mainly on non-keratinised mucosa
    (b) Usually present at the front of the mouth
    (c) Last up to two weeks in duration
    (d) Ulcers up to 3 cm in size
    (e) Heal without scarring

6. c

Acute pseudomembranous candidiasis is one of the most common forms of candidal infection. White plaques form and their removal reveals an erythematous background.

7. d

This is the only form of candidal infection that has a risk of becoming malignant. It usually forms a red/white patch that cannot be rubbed off. It is commonly seen in smokers, at the oral commissures, and biopsy is crucial.

8. b

Pemphigus is an example of type II hypersensitivity. Another example is pemphigoid.

9. d

Target lesions are common in erythema multiforme. This is often combined with oral lesions and ocular problems. It is commonly an acute type III hypersensitivity reaction and can occur in response to medications. Treatment usually involves a short course of steroids.

10. d

Ulcers in minor RAS tend to be smaller (up to 1 cm) in size. Larger ulcers are a more common feature of major RAS.

11. Shilling's test can be used to diagnose which of the following deficiencies?
(a) Iron
(b) Folate
(c) Vitamin B12
(d) Vitamin C
(e) Vitamin D

12. What is the peak incidence age for erythema multiforme?
(a) 10–15 years
(b) 10–20 years
(c) 20–30 years
(d) 30–40 years
(e) 40–50 years

13. Which of the following is not a precancerous condition?
(a) Actinic keratosis
(b) Lichen planus
(c) Submucous fibrosis
(d) Chronic hyperplastic candidiasis
(e) Pemphigus

14. A 14-year-old presents with bilateral, painful enlargement of the parotid glands. What is the likely diagnosis?
(a) Mumps
(b) Bacterial sialadenitis
(c) Recurrent parotitis
(d) Radiation sialadenitis
(e) Parotid abscess

15. Where do mucous extravasation cysts most commonly occur?
(a) Hard palate
(b) Soft palate
(c) Upper lip
(d) Lower lip
(e) Tongue

11. c

Shilling's test can be done to identify vitamin B12 deficiency. Fasting is required before the test and involves administration of radiolabelled vitamin B12, with further monitoring.

12. c

Peak incidence for erythema multiforme is usually 20–30 years of age. It usually has an acute onset and lasts around 2–3 weeks.

13. e

A precancerous condition is a generalised state associated with an increased risk of cancer development. Pemphigus is not associated with cancer development.

14. a

This childhood infection is caused by a paramyxovirus and is prevented by the MMR vaccine. Bacterial sialadenitis will generally present as a unilateral swelling.

15. d

Mucous extravasation cysts commonly occur due to trauma to the lower lip. They are often found in younger patients and they may recur. Mucous retention cysts tend to occur in older patients due to blockage of salivary ducts.

16. Which of the following unstimulated salivary flow rates would indicate a problem?
   (a) <1.5 mL in 5 minutes
   (b) <5 mL in 5 minutes
   (c) <1.5 mL in 15 minutes
   (d) <5 mL in 15 minutes
   (e) <0.5 mL in 15 minutes

17. Which of the following is not strongly associated with human immunodeficiency virus (HIV) infection?
   (a) Candidiasis
   (b) Hairy leukoplakia
   (c) Kaposi's sarcoma
   (d) Linear gingival erythema
   (e) Melanotic hyperpigmentation

18. Kaposi's sarcoma is associated with which virus?
   (a) HHV4
   (b) HHV7
   (c) HHV8
   (d) HHV1
   (e) HHV5

19. Which of the following is a symptom of trigeminal neuralgia?
   (a) Brief stabbing pain
   (b) Long-lasting stabbing pain
   (c) Affecting branches of the facial nerve
   (d) Short aching pain
   (e) Long-lasting ache

20. What is the first-line drug of choice for trigeminal neuralgia?
   (a) Phenytoin
   (b) Paracetamol
   (c) Valproate
   (d) Baclofen
   (e) Carbamazepine

16. c

This would indicate reduced function. For a stimulated salivary flow rate, anything less than 5 mL in 5 minutes would indicate reduced function.

17. e

Melanotic hyperpigmentation is only possibly associated with HIV. The other conditions are all strongly associated and are often first presentations of these patients.

18. c

HHV8 is responsible for Kaposi's sarcoma development. It most commonly presents on the hard palate and the gingivae, often looking similar to a pyogenic granuloma.

19. a

Trigeminal neuralgia is characterised by a brief stabbing pain. It is typically unilateral and in the distribution of the trigeminal nerve. The mandibular branch is the most commonly impacted branch.

20. e

Carbamazepine is the usual drug of choice for trigeminal neuralgia. It is a sodium channel blocker. The other drugs are potential options for pain management.

21. Which blood test should be done to monitor the drug in Question 20?
  (a) Platelet count
  (b) Full blood count
  (c) Liver function tests
  (d) B12 levels
  (e) Iron levels

22. Temporal arteritis will lead to which of the following if left untreated?
  (a) Blindness
  (b) Deafness
  (c) Long-term headache
  (d) Tinnitus
  (e) Blocked nose

23. Which of the following is not seen in Gorlin–Goltz syndrome?
  (a) Multiple basal cell carcinomas
  (b) Multiple odontogenic keratocysts
  (c) Calcification of the falx cerebri
  (d) Multiple squamous cell carcinomas
  (e) Frontal bossing

24. Which of the following is not typical of white sponge naevus?
  (a) Bilateral presentation
  (b) Lifelong
  (c) Family history
  (d) Malignant change
  (e) Thick white folds

25. Squamous cell papillomas are commonly caused by which virus?
  (a) HPV
  (b) HIV
  (c) EBV
  (d) HSV
  (e) HEV

21. c

Liver function tests are required because carbamazapine is metabolised by the liver and can impact its function. It may even lead to inflammation of the liver (hepatitis).

22. a

Temporal arteritis can lead to damage to the ophthalmic artery and subsequent ischaemia of the retina, hence causing blindness. Urgent steroids are required to minimise the impact to the eye.

23. d

Squamous cell carcinomas are not associated with Gorlin–Goltz syndrome.

24. d

White sponge naevus is not typically associated with malignant change; however, it often runs in families and has been present throughout life.

25. a

Human papillomavirus is commonly associated with the development of squamous cell papillomas. These are commonly found on the palate as a white cauliflower-like growth.

26. Syphilis is caused by which of the following bacteria?
    (a) *Treponema denticola*
    (b) *Treponema pallidum*
    (c) *Treponema vincentii*
    (d) *Prevotella intermedia*
    (e) *Fusobacterium necrophorum*

27. Which of the following would be prescribed to a patient suffering from shingles?
    (a) Metronidazole
    (b) Aciclovir
    (c) Amoxicillin
    (d) Fusidic acid
    (e) Tetracycline

28. Which of the following is a prodromal sign of a measles infection?
    (a) Koplik's spots
    (b) Wickham's striae
    (c) Epithelial hyperplasia
    (d) Target lesions
    (e) Nikolsky's sign

29. A 56-year-old female patient presents with several well-marginated ulcers, fiery red gingivae and conjunctivitis. Her skin appears clear. What is the likely diagnosis?
    (a) Pemphigus vulgaris
    (b) Bullous pemphigoid
    (c) Mucous membrane pemphigoid
    (d) Erythema multiforme
    (e) Crohn's disease

30. Which of the following is not a form of lichen planus?
    (a) Bullous
    (b) Ulcerative
    (c) Atrophic
    (d) Hypertrophic
    (e) Reticular

26. b

Treponema pallidum is the causative organism for syphilis. The infection is comprised of a primary, secondary and rarely a tertiary stage.

27. b

Shingles is due to reactivation of the varicella zoster virus and so only antivirals would be suitable to manage this.

28. a

Koplik's spots are seen in the prodromal phase of a measles infection. They are usually found on the buccal mucosae and are small white spots surrounded by a red ring.

29. c

This is most probably mucous membrane pemphigoid presenting with desquamative gingivitis, eye signs and ulcers. Bullous pemphigoid typically also presents with skin lesions.

30. d

Lichen planus has a hyperplastic form but not a hypertrophic form.

31. Which of the following is a high-risk site for oral cancer?
  (a) Lateral border of the tongue
  (b) Hard palate
  (c) Gingivae
  (d) Labial mucosa
  (e) Buccal mucosa

32. A 20-year-old man presents with a buccal swelling associated with his partially erupted wisdom tooth. Which of the following cysts is this most likely to be?
  (a) Odontogenic keratocyst
  (b) Paradental cyst
  (c) Dentigerous cyst
  (d) Gingival cyst
  (e) Glandular odontogenic cyst

33. A four-year-old boy presents with a mild fever and ulcers/vesicles on his soft palate. There is nothing else significant to note. What is he most likely suffering from?
  (a) Hand, foot and mouth
  (b) Measles
  (c) Herpangina
  (d) Glandular fever
  (e) Cold sores

34. What is the cause of the infection in Question 33?
  (a) Herpes simplex
  (b) Coxsackie A
  (c) Coxsackie B
  (d) Human papillomavirus
  (e) Epstein–Barr virus

31. a

The high-risk sites for oral cancer include floor of mouth, lateral borders of the tongue and the retromolar regions.

32. b

This is most probably a paradental cyst. They are most commonly associated with partially erupted wisdom teeth and present with inflammation from the periodontal pocket.

33. c

This is most likely herpangina. It is common in young patients with mild fever and ulcers and vesicles on the soft palate. It usually only lasts a few days and requires symptomatic management.

34. b

Herpangina is a Coxsackie A infection – typically A4.

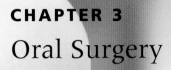

CHAPTER 3

Oral Surgery

Single Best Answer Questions for Dentistry, First Edition. Prateek Biyani.
© 2021 John Wiley & Sons Ltd. Published 2021 by John Wiley & Sons Ltd.

1. What is maximum dosage of paracetamol in a 24-hour period?
   (a) 1 g
   (b) 2 g
   (c) 4 g
   (d) 8 g
   (e) 10 g

2. Which is the most common reason for extraction of wisdom teeth?
   (a) Incisor crowding
   (b) Dentigerous cyst
   (c) Resorption
   (d) Periodontal pocketing
   (e) Pericoronitis

3. Which complication would not occur following extraction of lower wisdom teeth?
   (a) Trismus
   (b) Lingual nerve damage
   (c) Pain
   (d) Inferior alveolar nerve damage
   (e) Fractured tuberosity

4. Which of the following is not appropriate management for an unerupted tooth?
   (a) No treatment
   (b) Operculectomy
   (c) Surgically expose
   (d) Surgically remove
   (e) Removal of obstruction

5. What must be checked prior to extraction on a patient taking warfarin?
   (a) Platelet levels
   (b) FBCs
   (c) INR
   (d) LFTs
   (e) Thrombin time

1. c

The general dosage for paracetamol is 500 mg–1 g QDS, with a maximum 4 g dosage in 24 hours.

2. e

Pericoronitis, inflammation surrounding the crown of a partially erupted tooth, is the most common cause for extraction of wisdom teeth.

3. e

Fractured tuberosities would be a potential complication of an upper extraction, not a lower.

4. b

Operculectomy is not appropriate management for an unerupted tooth. It may be suitable for a partially erupted tooth.

5. c

A patient's INR must be checked if they are taking warfarin. This should ideally be below 4 prior to any dental procedures.

6. Which clotting factors does warfarin inhibit?
   (a) I, II, III, IV
   (b) II, V, IV, X
   (c) II, VII, IX, X
   (d) II, VI, IX, X
   (e) I, VII, IX, X

7. Which of the following may leave a patient prone to medication-related osteonecrosis of the jaw (MRONJ)?
   (a) Radiotherapy
   (b) Pamidronate
   (c) Metronidazole
   (d) Dabigatran
   (e) Rivaroxaban

8. When would an incisional biopsy most probably be used?
   (a) Squamous cell carcinoma
   (b) Papilloma
   (c) Polyp
   (d) Mucocoele
   (e) Amalgam tattoo

9. Which of the following methods is most commonly used to close an oro-antral communication (OAC)?
   (a) Buccal rotation flap
   (b) Palatal advancement flap
   (c) Palatal rotation flap
   (d) Buccal advancement flap
   (e) Buccal repositioned flap

10. What is the management of a squamous cell papilloma?
   (a) Radiotherapy
   (b) Chemotherapy
   (c) Simple excision with margins
   (d) Surgical removal plus neck dissection
   (e) Antibiotics

6. c

Warfarin inhibits clotting factors II, VII, IX and X.

7. b

Pamidronate is an example of a bisphosphonate and, therefore, is associated with MRONJ. Extractions should ideally be avoided in patients who are taking bisphosphonates due to risk of poor or incomplete healing.

8. a

All other lesions can be removed using excisional biopsies. An incisional biopsy should be used for an SCC to ensure proper treatment can be carried out afterwards.

9. d

Buccal advancement flaps are most commonly used to close OACs. Palatal rotation flaps can sometimes be used but are less successful, particularly due to a compromised blood supply.

10. c

Squamous cell papillomas are not of major concern and simple excision is required. They are caused by the human papillomavirus.

11. Which of the following is not a sign of Ludwig's angina?
(a) Difficulty breathing
(b) Dysphagia
(c) Cellulitis in submandibular area
(d) Odynophagia
(e) Facial nerve palsy

12. Which nerve provides motor innervation to the tongue?
(a) Facial nerve
(b) Lingual nerve
(c) Hypoglossal nerve
(d) Inferior alveolar nerve
(e) Maxillary nerve

13. Which strains of the human papillomavirus are thought to be associated with oral cancer?
(a) 1 and 2
(b) 4 and 8
(c) 12 and 14
(d) 16 and 18
(e) 18 and 20

14. Which of the following would characterise non-homogenous leukoplakia?
(a) Uniform
(b) Flat
(c) Plaque-like
(d) Single colour
(e) Speckled

15. Which of the following would not be a red flag for a cancerous lymph node?
(a) Soft swelling
(b) Painless
(c) Solid node
(d) Fixed tissues
(e) Rapid enlargement

11. e

Ludwig's angina describes life-threatening infection spreading in the submandibular area. Airway management, IV antibiotics and surgical drainage are usually required.

12. c

The hypoglossal nerve, cranial nerve XII, is responsible for motor supply to the tongue. Sensory innervation comes from the lingual, facial and glossopharyngeal nerves.

13. d

Strains 16 and 18 are thought to be strongly associated with development of oral cancer.

14. e

Non-homogenous leukoplakias appear abnormal and are often a combination of red and white regions. They may be exophytic and speckled. They have a higher risk of becoming malignant compared to homogenous leukoplakia.

15. a

Generally, a solid, painless enlarging lymph node is a red flag. Fixation would usually indicate extracapsular spread from the node into surrounding tissues.

16. Which N classification, of the TNM system, would indicate spread to a single ipsilateral lymph node of dimensions between 3 and 6 cm?
(a) N1
(b) N2a
(c) N2b
(d) N2c
(e) N3

17. Which of the following would not normally increase a patient's risk of bleeding?
(a) Warfarin
(b) Aspirin
(c) Dabigatran
(d) Apixaban
(e) Paracetamol

18. In which salivary gland are calculi most commonly found?
(a) Parotid
(b) Submandibular
(c) Sublingual
(d) Palatal
(e) Buccal

19. Which of the following methods is not used for calculi management?
(a) Basket removal
(b) Lithotripsy
(c) Surgical removal
(d) Conservative management
(e) Radiotherapy

20. Which of the following describes a condition causing gustatory sweating?
(a) Gorlin's syndrome
(b) Frey's syndrome
(c) Heart's syndrome
(d) Shell's syndrome
(e) Freid's syndrome

16. b

N2a indicates spread to a single ipsilateral lymph node with a size of between 3 and 6 cm.

17. e

All the other drugs increase a patient's risk of bleeding. Dabigatran and apixaban are both examples of novel oral anticoagulants.

18. b

The submandibular gland is most commonly affected by calculi. One of the reasons for this is thought to be because of the bend of the gland and duct around the mylohyoid muscle.

19. e

Radiotherapy is never used for management of salivary calculi. Conservative management is often sufficient.

20. b

Frey's syndrome often occurs following surgery in the parotid region. It occurs due to cross-innervation of nerves.

21. What is the most effective way of attempting to treat trigeminal neuralgia surgically?
    (a) Cryoanalgesia
    (b) Radiosurgery
    (c) Microvascular decompression
    (d) Glycerol injection
    (e) Thermocoagulation

22. Which of the following techniques is commonly used to remove odontogenic keratocysts in order to minimise damage to surrounding structures?
    (a) Vorschmidt's
    (b) Verschmit's
    (c) Malhart's
    (d) Hilton's
    (e) Hatton's

23. What is the general method of management for ameloblastomas?
    (a) Enucleation
    (b) Marsupialisation
    (c) Surgical resection
    (d) Curettage
    (e) Ablation

24. Where does the mandibular condyle sit at rest in the temporomandibular joint?
    (a) Articular eminence
    (b) Zygomatic arch
    (c) Glenoid fossa
    (d) Mastoid notch
    (e) Sigmoid notch

25. What imaging would initially be requested for a fractured mandible?
    (a) OPT and bitewings
    (b) OPT and PA mandible
    (c) PA mandible + OM view
    (d) Two OM Views
    (e) OPT and CT Scan

21. c

Microvascular decompression is thought to be the most effective way in fit and healthy patients. Other methods provide limited improvement for patients, but may be the only suitable methods.

22. a

This involves fixing the cyst prior to enucleation using Carnoy's solution. This aims to allow for complete removal of the cyst with minimal damage to surrounding structures, particularly the inferior alveolar nerve.

23. c

Generally, surgical resection is necessary for ameloblastomas. It is only in true unicystic ameloblastomas where enucleation may be carried out.

24. c

The glenoid fossa in the temporal bone is where the mandibular condyle normally sits.

25. b

The first line of imaging for a fractured mandible is typically an OPT and a PA mandible. Two views from different angles allow for better visualisation of the fracture.

26. Which of the following surgical methods is often used for a simple fractured zygoma?
    (a) Caldwell–Luc incision
    (b) Smith's lift
    (c) Gilles approach
    (d) Gunning approach
    (e) Millard's approach

27. What would be given to a patient suffering from Haemophilia A?
    (a) Factor VII concentrate
    (b) Factor IX concentrate
    (c) Factor V concentrate
    (d) Factor VIII concentrate
    (e) Factor X concentrate

28. Which of the following is a novel oral anticoagulant?
    (a) Warfarin
    (b) Heparin
    (c) Aspirin
    (d) Clopidogrel
    (e) Apixaban

29. Which instrument is used to dilate and detach the periodontal ligament prior to an extraction?
    (a) Couplands
    (b) Luxator
    (c) Warwick James
    (d) Cryers
    (e) Forceps

30. A patient presents with a swelling over the angle of the mandible. He has been suffering from a fever and feels quite unwell. What are you likely to prescribe?
    (a) Nothing
    (b) Amoxicillin 200 mg TDS
    (c) Metronidazole 250 mg BD
    (d) Amoxicillin 500 mg TDS
    (e) Metronidazole 450 mg TDS

26. c

The Gilles approach is often used to reduce the zygoma back into position. It involves an incision near the temple, identifying the temporalis muscle and following this under the zygoma.

27. d

Haemophilia A is a deficiency in factor VIII. As a result, a patient may be given factor VIII concentrate to minimise their bleeding risk.

28. e

Apixaban is one of the novel oral anticoagulants. Others include dabigatran and rivaroxaban.

29. b

Luxators are commonly used to gently detach the PDL and widen the socket before applying forceps.

30. d

This patient has systemic involvement and requires antibiotics. Amoxicillin and metronidazole are the two main antibiotics to consider. Only **d** has the correct dosage.

31. Which biopsy technique should be used to assess a white patch of unknown origin?
  (a) Excisional biopsy
  (b) Fine needle aspirate
  (c) Incisional biopsy
  (d) Core needle biopsy
  (e) Ethyl chloride

32. Metronidazole is known to cause disulfiram-like reactions. In which group of patients is this likely to occur?
  (a) Asthmatics
  (b) Patients allergic to latex
  (c) Alcoholics
  (d) Smokers
  (e) Patients taking amoxicillin

33. Which of the following would not increase the risk of fracturing a mandible whilst extracting a tooth?
  (a) Atrophic mandible
  (b) Large, bony defect
  (c) Existing bone pathology
  (d) Dense bone
  (e) Use of excessive force

34. What is the approximate percentage risk of permanent lingual nerve injury from third molar removal?
  (a) 5%
  (b) 10%
  (c) 7%
  (d) 0.5%
  (e) 1.5%

35. Which of the following is not an advantage of laser surgery?
  (a) No tactile sensation
  (b) Precision
  (c) Reduced haemorrhage
  (d) Rapid incision
  (e) No touch

31. c

An incisional biopsy should be used to ensure a sample of healthy and diseased tissue is taken. This will allow for better assessment of the lesion.

32. c

Metronidazole and alcohol have a significant interaction and should be completely avoided. Any patient must be warned not to consume alcohol if they are to be given metronidazole. It will lead to nausea, vomiting and other potential systemic issues.

33. d

Dense bone is less likely to lead to a fractured mandible on its own – though it may make the extraction more difficult. Atrophic mandibles, particularly in elderly, osteoporotic patients, are particularly high risk.

34. d

Around 0.5% of lingual nerve injuries will be permanent following wisdom tooth removal.

35. a

There is a lack of tactile sensation when attempting to carry out laser surgery. The lack of touch at the surgical site reduces the risk of infection.

CHAPTER 4

Oral Pathology

Single Best Answer Questions for Dentistry, First Edition. Prateek Biyani.
© 2021 John Wiley & Sons Ltd. Published 2021 by John Wiley & Sons Ltd.

1. Which of the following is observed in white sponge naevus?
   (a) Loss of epithelium
   (b) Inflammation
   (c) Orthokeratin
   (d) Acanthosis
   (e) Tzank cells

2. Which condition is caused by autoantibodies against desmoglein 3?
   (a) Pemphigus foliaceous
   (b) Pemphigus vulgaris
   (c) Mucous membrane pemphigoid
   (d) Bullous pemphigoid
   (e) Dermatitis herpetiformis

3. Which key inflammatory cell is noted in oral lichen planus?
   (a) B cell
   (b) T cell
   (c) Macrophage
   (d) Neutrophil
   (e) IgD

4. What pattern is observed when direct immunofluorescence is carried out on a pemphigus biopsy?
   (a) Fishnet
   (b) Straight line
   (c) Circular
   (d) Web
   (e) Bubble

5. Which of the following characterises an ulcer?
   (a) Fluid infiltrate
   (b) Partial loss of epithelium
   (c) Complete break in the epithelium
   (d) Increase in epithelial thickness
   (e) Increased iron deposition

1. d

White sponge naevus is typically uninflamed but is characterised by acanthosis, an increased thickness of the prickle cell layer of the epithelium.

2. b

Pemphigus vulgaris is characterised by autoantibodies targeting the desmosomes within the epithelium.

3. b

There is the presence of a marked T-cell band in lichen planus, as it is a type IV hypersensitivity response. These can be seen below the basement membrane.

4. a

A characteristic fishnet appearance is seen due to the presence of autoantibodies present at desmosomes between cells. This is different from pemphigoid, where fluorescence occurs at the basement membrane.

5. c

Ulcers are characterised by having a complete loss of overlying epithelium. Partial thickness loss refers to an erosive lesion, which often takes longer to heal.

6. Which of the following is not described as being a dysplastic change?
   (a) Irregular mitosis
   (b) Loss of epithelial stratification
   (c) Basal cell hyperplasia
   (d) Presence of a prickle cell layer
   (e) Loss of intercellular adherence

7. What percentage of non-homogenous leukoplakia lesions progress to malignancy?
   (a) 0%
   (b) 5%
   (c) 20%
   (d) 50%
   (e) 80%

8. Which of the following features indicates a poor prognosis with oral cancer?
   (a) Well-differentiated cells
   (b) Well-localised lesion
   (c) Non-cohesive invasion
   (d) Minimal depth of invasion
   (e) No involvement of other structures

9. Which of the following features is not usually seen with salivary calculi?
   (a) Chronic inflammatory cells
   (b) Fibrous septa
   (c) Acinar cell destruction
   (d) Duct dilation
   (e) Civatte bodies

10. Regarding mucous extravasation cysts, which of the following is false?
    (a) They most commonly occur on the lower lip
    (b) They are more common in older people
    (c) They are typically associated with a history of trauma
    (d) They are the most common type of mucocoele
    (e) They may recur

6. d

A prickle cell layer is a normal component of epithelium and is not a dysplastic change. Dysplasia refers to cellular and architectural change within the tissue, including abnormal mitosis and loss of stratification.

7. c

This is higher than homogenous leukoplakia which lies more around 5%.

8. c

Non-cohesive invasion indicates that islands of invading epithelium have spread as they have invaded. This makes it difficult to fully resect the cancer as well as increasing the risk of metastasis.

9. e

Civatte bodies are characteristic of lichen planus.

10. b

Mucous extravasation cysts are most commonly found in younger patients due to their association with trauma. They do not possess a proper epithelial lining as often the salivary duct is damaged. They may recur due to the nature of their origin.

11. Which of the following is the most common salivary gland neoplasm?
    (a) Adenoid cystic carcinoma
    (b) Mucoepidermoid carcinoma
    (c) Pleomorphic adenoma
    (d) Warthin's tumour
    (e) Basal cell adenoma

12. Adenoid cystic carcinomas are characterised by what appearance?
    (a) Swiss cheese
    (b) Thread-like
    (c) Capsulated
    (d) Myxoid
    (e) Monotonous

13. Which of the following lesions typically demonstrates pigment along collagen fibres and around blood vessels?
    (a) Malignant melanoma
    (b) Post-inflammatory lesions
    (c) Amalgam tattoo
    (d) Black hairy tongue
    (e) Naevus

14. Which of the following develops from the reduced enamel epithelium?
    (a) Radicular cysts
    (b) Keratocysts
    (c) Gingival cysts
    (d) Dentigerous cysts
    (e) Nasopalatine cysts

15. Which of the following is not a developmental odontogenic cyst?
    (a) Paradental cyst
    (b) Odontogenic keratocyst
    (c) Gingival cyst
    (d) Dentigerous cyst
    (e) Eruption cyst

11. c

Pleomorphic adenomas account for nearly 70% of salivary gland neoplasms. They are generally benign but may become malignant in the long term, so excision is often the best management option.

12. a

Adenoid cystic carcinomas lack a capsule and have a multicystic appearance – this leads to a 'Swiss cheese', or cribriform, appearance.

13. c

Amalgam tattoos typically present like this. They often present as flat, greyish lesions along the alveolar ridges. They can be diagnosed using a radiograph or biopsy.

14. d

Radicular cysts develop from the cell rests of Malassez, while keratocysts and gingival cysts develop from the dental lamina.

15. a

Paradental cysts are typically associated with inflammation surrounding partially erupted wisdom teeth.

16. Radicular cysts may contain all of the following except:
    (a) Cholesterol
    (b) Keratin
    (c) Hyaline bodies
    (d) Mucous cells
    (e) Serous cells

17. Which type of epithelium is found in odontogenic keratocysts?
    (a) Thick stratified squamous epithelium
    (b) Thin simple squamous epithelium
    (c) Thin parakeratinised stratified squamous epithelium
    (d) Thin orthokeratinised stratified squamous epithelium
    (e) Thick parakeratinised stratified cuboidal epithelium

18. Which of the following is not a form of ameloblastoma?
    (a) Plexiform
    (b) Unicystic
    (c) Follicular
    (d) Peripheral
    (e) Multicentric

19. Which of the following, regarding odontomes, is not true?
    (a) They are hamartomas
    (b) They may prevent eruption of teeth
    (c) They are potentially malignant
    (d) They generally occur in younger patients
    (e) They can present in both the mandible and maxilla

20. Osteomas are associated with which syndrome?
    (a) Albright's
    (b) Grave's
    (c) Gardner's
    (d) Cushing's
    (e) Down's

16. e

Serous cells are not seen in radicular cysts.

17. c

Odontogenic keratocysts are characterised by a thin parakeratinised stratified squamous epithelium that lacks rete ridges.

18. e

The most common are solid ameloblastomas which include follicular and plexiform types. Ameloblastomas typically require resection with margins due to their risk of recurrence. Unicystic ameloblastomas may be treated like a normal cyst.

19. c

Odontomes are not associated with malignancies. They are hamartomas which may be complex or compound in nature.

20. c

Patients with Gardner's syndrome develop multiple intestinal polyps as well as jaw osteomas.

21. Which of the following best describes an ossifying fibroma?
   (a) A reactive lesion with irregular trabecular of woven bone and cementum
   (b) A benign neoplasm with fibrous tissue and islands of bone
   (c) A developmental lesion with irregular trabecular of woven bone and cementum
   (d) A reactive lesion with cementum and bone only
   (e) A malignant neoplasm showing aggressive invasion

22. Fibrous dysplasia can be differentiated from ossifying fibromas on biopsies because:
   (a) Fibrous dysplasia is well-defined relative to ossifying fibromas
   (b) Fibrous dysplasia is more common in the mandible
   (c) Fibrous dysplasia has a clear margin
   (d) Fibrous dysplasia is a poorly-defined lesion relative to ossifying fibromas
   (e) Ossifying fibromas are more common in males

23. Which of the following is a tumour of odontogenic epithelium only?
   (a) Odontome
   (b) Myxoma
   (c) Ameloblastic fibroma
   (d) Ameloblastoma
   (e) Cementoblastoma

24. Which of the following is a non-odontogenic cyst?
   (a) Nasolabial cyst
   (b) Radicular cyst
   (c) Dentigerous cyst
   (d) Residual cyst
   (e) Gingival cyst

25. Which of the following shows an increased thickness of keratin with a papilliferous outline and a surface thrown into fronds?
   (a) Erythroplakia
   (b) Aphthous ulcer
   (c) Squamous cell papilloma
   (d) White sponge naevus
   (e) Chronic hyperplastic candidiasis

21. b

Ossifying fibromas are benign neoplasms which occur most commonly in the mandible and in females.

22. d

Although fibrous dysplasia is a developmental lesion, it is often poorly-defined with no clear margins. This makes it more difficult to manage and remove. As the lesions are developmental, management can be considered once growth has ceased.

23. d

Odontomes and ameloblastic fibromas develop from both odontogenic epithelium and mesenchyme, whilst the other tumours are mesenchyme only.

24. a

Nasolabial and nasopalatine cysts are the most common non-odontogenic cysts that are seen.

25. c

Squamous cell papillomas appear as white, 'wart-like' lesions typically on the palate. They appear white due to the increase in keratin. They are usually caused by the human papillomavirus.

26. Which of the following shows a band-like accumulation of T cells below the basement membrane and saw-tooth rete ridges?
(a) Erythema multiforme
(b) Lichen planus
(c) Leukoplakia
(d) Chronic hyperplastic candidiasis
(e) White sponge naevus

27. Which of the following is not an autoimmune condition?
(a) Lichen planus
(b) Dermatitis herpetiformis
(c) Epidermolysis bullosa congenita
(d) Pemphigus vulgaris
(e) Bullous pemphigoid

28. Which of the following would not reduce the healing ability of a patient?
(a) Immunosuppression
(b) Chemotherapy
(c) Good blood supply
(d) Irradiation
(e) Nutritional deficiency

29. Which of the following is not a recognised component of the developing enamel organ?
(a) Stratum intermedium
(b) Stellate reticulum
(c) Primary epithelial band
(d) Internal dental epithelium
(e) External dental epithelium

26. b

Lichen planus is a cell-mediated type IV reaction demonstrating a band-like accumulation of T cells below the basement membrane.

27. c

Epidermolysis bullosa congenita is an inherited condition which affects the proteins in the epithelium and connective tissue. These are usually proteins required for anchoring.

28. c

A good blood supply would ensure that healing could occur properly. Irradiation can reduce blood supply, whilst the other options may make a patient more susceptible to infection and reduced healing.

29. c

The primary epithelial band is one of the first signs of tooth development and represents a thickened band of ectoderm. The enamel organ forms later in the development process and is made up of the other four layers.

30. What is the name given to the rod-like structures observed within bone?
   (a) Compact bone
   (b) Haversian systems
   (c) Volkmann's canals
   (d) Osteoid
   (e) Trabeculae

31. Which cells are responsible for dentine formation and deposition?
   (a) Odontoblasts
   (b) Osteoblasts
   (c) Odontoclasts
   (d) Osteocytes
   (e) Ameloblasts

30. e

Trabeculae make up 'rods' within the cancellous bone and allow for weight bearing. Compact bone lines the outside. Volkmann's canals travel into Haversian systems to allow nutrients and blood vessels access. Osteoid refers to the first organic matrix secreted by osteoblasts – this is later calcified.

31. a

Osteoblasts, osteoclasts and osteocytes are cells involved in bone formation, resorption and regulation respectively. Ameloblasts are responsible for enamel deposition and maturation.

CHAPTER 5

Paediatric Dentistry and Orthodontics

1. Which of the following injuries best describes 'injury to the supporting tooth tissues without displacement'?
   (a) Luxation
   (b) Avulsion
   (c) Subluxation
   (d) Concussion
   (e) Extrusion

2. What is the maximum dosage of fluoride that a 12-year-old child could safely have in their toothpaste?
   (a) 500 ppm
   (b) 1000 ppm
   (c) 1350 ppm
   (d) 2800 ppm
   (e) 5000 ppm

3. In which of the following situations is a Hall crown strictly contraindicated?
   (a) Pulpal involvement
   (b) Multi-surface caries
   (c) Needle-phobic patients
   (d) Trauma
   (e) Asymptomatic tooth

4. A child presents with an overjet of 8 mm and contact point displacements of 3 mm. What would their Index of Orthodontic Treatment Need (IOTN) category be?
   (a) 3d
   (b) 3a
   (c) 4a
   (d) 4b
   (e) 5a

5. Which of the following is not an indication of non-accidental injury (NAI)?
   (a) Delay in seeking treatment
   (b) Withdrawn child
   (c) History matching presentation
   (d) Trauma in 'safe zones'
   (e) Poor interaction between parent and child

1. d

Subluxation would involve loosening of the tooth without displacement, whilst luxation would involve some type of displacement. The more significant the trauma, the poorer the prognosis of the pulp.

2. d

A prescription toothpaste of 2800 ppm fluoride is the maximum a child of this age may be given. Children over the age of 16 may receive 5000 ppm.

3. a

Any sign of pulpal involvement contraindicates placement of a Hall crown. In the right situation, a Hall crown is an excellent evidence-based method of caries management. The lack of local anaesthetic and preparation required is perfect for less co-operative children.

4. c

4a refers to an overjet between 6.1 and 9 mm. 5a would be anything above this. Although the contact point displacement is a 3d, it is lower in the IOTN scale compared to an overjet.

5. c

NAI may be suspected when the history does not match the clinical presentation of the child.

6. Extrusion is defined by which of the following?
   (a) Injury to tooth-supporting structures without an increase in mobility or displacement
   (b) Displacement of a tooth in a direction other than the axial direction
   (c) Displacement of a tooth completely out of its socket
   (d) Partial displacement of a tooth out of its socket
   (e) Increased mobility but no displacement

7. Which of the following would not be an indication for extracting a deciduous tooth?
   (a) Risk of bleeding
   (b) Unrestorable tooth
   (c) Acute infection
   (d) Extensive associated pathology
   (e) Immunosuppresion

8. A child presents with hypomineralised, broken down first permanent molars and a white lesion on his UR1. What is the likely diagnosis?
   (a) Fluorosis
   (b) Turner tooth
   (c) Molar-incisor hypomineralisation (MIH)
   (d) Caries
   (e) Tetracycline staining

9. What would generally be prescribed to a routinely healthy child presenting with a primary herpes infection?
   (a) Aciclovir
   (b) Penicillin
   (c) Metronidazole
   (d) Nystatin
   (e) Paracetamol

10. Which of the following conditions would present with amber discolouration, bulbous crowns and pulpal obliteration?
   (a) Amelogenesis imperfecta (AI)
   (b) MIH
   (c) Dentinogenesis imperfecta (DI)
   (d) Down's syndrome
   (e) Taurodontism

6. d

b describes lateral luxation compared to extrusion.

7. a

Immunosuppression may mean the patient will not be able to manage any residual infection and so an extraction may be indicated in this situation.

8. c

The first permanent molars can often be referred to as 'cheesy molars'. MIH affects at least one of the four first permanent molars and may affect incisors. The teeth tend to be very sensitive and difficult to anaesthetise, making management very difficult. A Turner tooth is consequent to trauma/infection in a deciduous tooth impacting the developing permanent tooth. It would not be as widespread as this.

9. e

Primary herpes is usually a self-limiting condition lasting only a few days. Supportive care, including analgesia such as paracetamol, is all that is necessary. Aciclovir is only required in more significant infections or in immunocompromised patients.

10. c

Patients with DI usually present with teeth that are lacking enamel and have exposed underlying dentine. The teeth also typically have narrow and short roots.

11. Patients with a cleft palate typically develop which type of malocclusion?
(a) Class I
(b) Class II Div 1
(c) Class II Div 2
(d) Class II intermediate
(e) Class III

12. Which of the following provides posterior retention in a removable appliance?
(a) Southend clasp
(b) C-clasp
(c) Labial arch
(d) Adams clasp
(e) Coffin spring

13. Which of the following refers to the 'lowermost point on the mandibular symphysis' in cephalometric analysis?
(a) Gonion
(b) Sella
(c) Nasion
(d) Menton
(e) B point

14. What is a balancing extraction?
(a) Extraction of the same tooth on the opposing arch on the same side
(b) Extraction of the same tooth on the opposing arch on the opposite side
(c) Extraction of the same tooth on the same arch on the opposite side
(d) Extraction of the same tooth from all quadrants
(e) Extraction of the same tooth on the opposing arch from both sides

15. Which of the following is not a known problem caused by digit sucking?
(a) Retroclined lower incisors
(b) Proclined upper incisors
(c) Anterior open bite
(d) Posterior crossbite
(e) Widening of upper arch

11. e

Patients with a cleft palate typically have poor growth of their maxilla which contributes to the development of a Class III malocclusion.

12. d

Adams clasps are usually placed on the first permanent molars. They provide retention, allow for attachments and provide a site for patients to apply pressure to remove the appliance.

13. d

Gonion is a constructed point, whilst sella refers to the pituitary fossa and nasion refers to the most anterior point of the frontonasal suture.

14. c

Balancing extractions may be done to avoid centreline shifts, particularly in deciduous teeth. **a** refers to a compensating extraction, which may be done to manage problems with overeruption.

15. e

The upper arch typically narrows due to digit sucking, thus creating a posterior crossbite.

16. Which of the following techniques/features would not be used to identify an ectopic canine?
    (a) Palpation
    (b) Radiography
    (c) Mobility of deciduous tooth
    (d) Angulation of lateral incisors
    (e) Tenderness to percussion

17. What would be the most appropriate management for a pinpoint exposure occurring only two hours ago following trauma?
    (a) Extraction
    (b) Root canal treatment
    (c) Direct pulp cap
    (d) Cvek pulpotomy
    (e) No specific management is needed

18. Which sedation agent is used for inhalation sedation?
    (a) Nitric oxide
    (b) Midazolam
    (c) Flumazenil
    (d) Nitrous oxide
    (e) Oxygen

19. Which of the following is not associated with hypodontia?
    (a) High birth weight
    (b) Increased maternal age
    (c) Single gene mutations
    (d) Down's syndrome
    (e) Ectodermal dysplasia

20. What should the angle (in degrees) for SNA be in cephalometric analysis?
    (a) 79 ± 1
    (b) 79 ± 3
    (c) 81 ± 3
    (d) 83 ± 3
    (e) 85 ± 1

16. e

Checking for tenderness to percussion would not provide any useful information regarding ectopic canines.

17. c

If the exposure occurred within 24 hours and is only pinpoint then a direct pulp cap is appropriate. However, if either of these parameters are not met then a Cvek pulpotomy is more appropriate.

18. d

Nitrous oxide is used for inhalation sedation. Nitrous oxide is very useful to sedate children and provide effective dental care. Midazolam is used for intravenous sedation, whilst flumazenil is midazolam's reversal agent.

19. a

Low birth weights are associated with hypodontia.

20. c

The typical value for SNA is 81 ± 3. These measurements are important in analysing a patient's skeletal class.

21. Which of the following behavioural management techniques involves demonstrating treatment on another family member or patient?
(a) Tell, show, do
(b) Modelling
(c) Positive reinforcement
(d) Negative reinforcement
(e) Desensitisation

22. Which of the following would be the most appropriate investigation(s) to locate an ectopic canine?
(a) Bitewing radiographs
(b) Orthopantomogram (OPG)
(c) OPG + periapical radiograph
(d) Periapical radiograph
(e) Lateral cephalogram + OPG

23. What best describes a complicated fracture of a tooth?
(a) A fracture extending through enamel
(b) A fracture extending through enamel and dentine without pulpal exposure
(c) A fracture extending through enamel, dentine and cementum without pulpal exposure
(d) A fracture extending through enamel and dentine with pulpal exposure
(e) A crack extending through enamel

24. Which of the following is the appropriate management for an avulsed primary tooth?
(a) Clean with chlorhexidine and reimplant
(b) Reimplant only if root is intact
(c) Reimplant immediately
(d) Do not reimplant
(e) Clean with saline and reimplant

25. What is the minimum toxic dose of fluoride?
(a) 1 mg/kg
(b) 2 mg/kg
(c) 3 mg/kg
(d) 4 mg/kg
(e) 5 mg/kg

21. b

Modelling is a good behavioural management technique helping to get children used to dental treatment and increase co-operation.

22. c

This will allow for the parallax technique and localisation of any ectopic canines. By assessing the movement of the canine between radiographs, you can assess whether the canine is buccally or palatally positioned. If the canine moves in the same direction as the tube then it is located palatally – otherwise it is located buccally.

23. d

Complicated fractures are those involving the pulp. Management depends upon the time of exposure, size of exposure and age of the patient.

24. d

An avulsed primary tooth should not be reimplanted due to the risk of damaging the permanent successor in the process.

25. e

Symptoms of fluoride toxicity include nausea, palpitations and breathlessness.

26. Down's syndrome is characterised by which genetic abnormality?
   (a) Trisomy 16
   (b) Trisomy 17
   (c) Trisomy 20
   (d) Trisomy 21
   (e) Trisomy 23

27. Which of the following could potentially be an abusive injury?
   (a) Graze on a child's knee
   (b) Bruise on a child's elbow
   (c) Bump on a child's forehead
   (d) Bruise behind a child's ear
   (e) Graze on a child's hand

28. Which of the following do functional appliances rely on?
   (a) Class I molars
   (b) Increased overbite
   (c) Active growth
   (d) Minimal growth
   (e) Non-motivated patient

29. Which of the following is a risk associated with early extraction of a lower first permanent molar?
   (a) Poor space closure
   (b) Mesial tipping of the second permanent molar
   (c) Second permanent molar leans buccally
   (d) Distal tipping of the second permanent molar
   (e) Second premolar drifts mesially

30. Which form of trauma in primary teeth is most likely to damage the secondary successor?
   (a) Subluxation
   (b) Concussion
   (c) Intrusion
   (d) Avulsion
   (e) Extrusion

26. d

Down's syndrome occurs due to an individual having three copies of chromosome 21. Patients with Down's syndrome can have multiple dental problems including hypodontia, microdontia and periodontal disease.

27. d

The area behind the ear and on to the neck is the 'triangle of safety'. This is an area that would not normally be accidentally injured. Therefore, injuries in this region should be treated with suspicion and the history should be investigated.

28. c

Functional appliances rely on active growth to help correct primarily Class II relationships, as well as sometimes Class III malocclusions.

29. b

Premature extraction of the first permanent molar causes the second permanent molar to tilt mesially and lean lingually. Early extraction would also cause the second permanent molar to drift distally.

30. c

Intrusion is most likely to damage the follicle of the developing secondary tooth. It is thought to affect the successor in up to 69% of cases. This is closely followed by avulsion.

31. Which of the following is not true regarding the differences between primary and secondary teeth?
(a) Primary teeth are smaller than secondary teeth
(b) Primary teeth have thicker enamel than secondary teeth
(c) Primary teeth have a larger pulp chamber than secondary teeth
(d) Contacts between primary posterior teeth are wider and flatter than secondary teeth
(e) Primary teeth have smaller roots than permanent teeth

32. What is the maximum dose of lignocaine that can be given as a local anaesthetic?
(a) 3.0 mg/kg
(b) 3.4 mg/kg
(c) 4.2 mg/kg
(d) 4.4 mg/kg
(e) 4.8 mg/kg

31. b

Primary teeth have thinner enamel than secondary teeth. All the factors discussed in this question make primary teeth more prone to caries and allow for rapid progression of caries. They often also make caries assessment more difficult.

32. d

The maximum dose of lignocaine that can be given is 4.4 mg/kg. This is crucial when considering local anaesthetic dosage for children and ensuring they are weighed and dosed accordingly.

CHAPTER 6

Periodontics

1. Which of the following form the 'red complex' organisms?
   (a) *Porphyromonas gingivalis, Fusobacterium necropharum, Treponema denticola*
   (b) *Shigella sonnei, Tannerella forsythia, Treponema denticola*
   (c) *Porphyromonas gingivalis, Shigella sonnei, Fusobacterium necropharum*
   (d) *Porphyromonas gingivalis, Tannerella forsythia, Treponema denticola*
   (e) *Prevotella intermedia, Tannerella forsythia, Treponema denticola*

2. How much pressure should be used when instrumenting with a Basic Periodontal Examination (BPE) probe?
   (a) 5 g
   (b) 10 g
   (c) 15 g
   (d) 20 g
   (e) 25 g

3. Which of the following is true with regards to gingivitis?
   (a) Changes are irreversible
   (b) There is alveolar bone destruction
   (c) Junctional epithelium remains attached at the amelocemental junction (ACJ)
   (d) It is managed through root surface debridement (RSD)
   (e) It is a rare condition

4. Which of the following is a sign of gingivitis?
   (a) Bleeding on probing
   (b) Stippled gingivae
   (c) No mobility
   (d) Normal probing depths
   (e) Plaque accumulation

5. Which of the following conditions is not associated with periodontitis?
   (a) Down's syndrome
   (b) Chediak–Higashi syndrome
   (c) Anaemia
   (d) Cohen syndrome
   (e) Hypophosphatasia

1. d

These are the red complex bacteria thought to be associated with development of periodontitis.

2. e

This is the precise amount of force – it is enough to make the skin under your nail blanch. Anything beyond this may damage the periodontal tissues.

3. c

Gingivitis is completely reversible with no loss of attachment or bone destruction. It is a very common condition amongst the population.

4. a

Bleeding is a common sign of gingivitis. Plaque, though not a sign of gingivitis, may be a common cause of its development.

5. c

Anaemia is not thought to be associated with development of periodontitis. All the other conditions are genetic disorders that are associated with it.

6. What does a BPE score of 3 indicate?
   (a) Pocketing between 3.5 and 5.5 mm
   (b) Pocketing over 5.5 mm
   (c) Pocketing less than 3.5 mm but plaque retentive features present
   (d) Bleeding upon probing
   (e) Furcation involvement

7. Which of the following is used to indicate furcation involvement in a BPE?
   (a) X
   (b) %
   (c) *
   (d) #
   (e) F

8. What is the appropriate management for a patient presenting with a BPE score of 3?
   (a) Oral hygiene instruction (OHI)
   (b) OHI and scaling
   (c) OHI, scaling and correction of plaque retentive features
   (d) OHI, scaling, full periodontal assessment and RSD
   (e) OHI, scaling, full periodontal assessment and gingival surgery

9. Which of the following probes is used to assess furcation involvement?
   (a) UNC-15
   (b) BPE
   (c) William's
   (d) Naber's
   (e) Marquis

10. What does a mobility score of Grade 2 indicate?
    (a) No mobility
    (b) Mobility in the horizontal direction <1 mm
    (c) Mobility in the horizontal direction 1–2 mm
    (d) Mobility in the vertical direction <1 mm
    (e) Mobility in the vertical direction 1–2 mm

6. a

A BPE of 3 indicates pocketing between 3.5 and 5.5 mm, which will mean the black band will be partially visible on a BPE probe.

7. c

An X is used where there is either one or no teeth in a sextant.

8. d

A full assessment should be completed and then RSD targeted at pockets which are 4 mm or more. This should then be reviewed in three months.

9. d

A Naber's probe is used to assess furcational involvement – it is divided into thirds which gives a score from F0 to F3.

10. c

Grading	Description
0	No mobility
1	Mobility in horizontal direction <1 mm
2	Mobility in horizontal direction 1–2 mm
3	Mobility in horizontal direction >2 mm or vertical mobility

11. Which radiograph would be indicated for a UR1 with 8 mm pockets?
(a) None
(b) Periapical
(c) Panoramic
(d) Upper standard occlusal (USO)
(e) Sectional panoramic

12. Which of the following is a local antimicrobial containing metronidazole?
(a) PerioChip®
(b) Atridox®
(c) Elyzol®
(d) Dentomycin®
(e) Chlosite®

13. Acute herpetic gingivostomatitis is caused by which of the following?
(a) Herpangina
(b) Herpes simplex I
(c) Varicella zoster
(d) HHV 8
(e) *Porphyromonas gingivalis*

14. Which of the following is seen in a lateral periodontal abscess but not in a periapical abscess?
(a) Non-vital tooth
(b) Apical change
(c) No history of periodontal disease
(d) Deep pocketing
(e) Extensive caries

15. Which of the following drugs is strongly associated with gingival overgrowth?
(a) Paracetamol
(b) Aspirin
(c) Ibuprofen
(d) Ciclosporin
(e) Warfarin

11. b

A periapical radiograph is the gold standard to assess bone levels in periodontal disease. A panoramic radiograph can sometimes be taken but the cervical spine would obscure the anterior teeth.

12. c

Elyzol® contains metronidazole and has been seen to be effective at managing certain periodontal diseases. PerioChip® (chlorhexidine), Dentomycin® (minocycline) and Atridox® (doxycycline) are all also local antimicrobials.

13. b

This is a viral infection and is the primary infection of herpes simplex I. It commonly presents with ulcers and vesicles in the mouth in younger patients.

14. d

All the other features would generally indicate a periapical abscess.

15. d

Ciclosporin is commonly associated with gingival overgrowth. Other drugs causing gingival overgrowth include phenytoin and amlodipine.

16. Which of the following is not a healthy feature of the gingivae?
    (a) Knife-edged margins
    (b) Light stippling
    (c) Smooth transition from gingiva to tooth
    (d) Presence of papilla
    (e) Recession

17. Which of the following is not an indication for periodontal surgery?
    (a) Removal of hyperplastic tissue
    (b) Correction of recession defects
    (c) Crown lengthening
    (d) Root surface debridement
    (e) Pocket elimination

18. Which of the following would be an indication for an apically repositioned flap?
    (a) Removal of hyperplastic tissue
    (b) Crown lengthening
    (c) Correction of recession defects
    (d) Implant placement
    (e) Correction of defects on adjacent teeth

19. Which of the following is not a complication following flap surgery?
    (a) Haemorrhage
    (b) Pain
    (c) Recession
    (d) Sensitivity
    (e) Reduced pocketing

20. Which of the following is not a precipitating factor for gingival recession?
    (a) Parafunctional habits
    (b) Food trauma
    (c) Thin cortical plate
    (d) Gingival inflammation
    (e) Toothbrushing trauma

16. e

Recession is generally a feature of disease, be it trauma or periodontal disease. This may be active or historic.

17. d

Root surface debridement is generally done without any periodontal surgery. This results in 'blind' cleaning of the root surface, which may not be sufficient.

18. b

Crown lengthening and pocket elimination are key indications for apically repositioned flaps.

19. e

A reduction in pocketing is a sign of successful surgery.

20. c

A thin cortical plate is a predisposing factor for development of gingival recession. This will then lead to recession when other precipitating factors are present.

21. Which of the following best describes *Treponema denticola*?
   (a) Gram-negative bacillus
   (b) Gram-positive spirochaete
   (c) Gram-negative spirochaete
   (d) Gram-positive bacillus
   (e) Gram-negative coccus

22. What percentage of plaque is formed by micro-organisms?
   (a) 30%
   (b) 50%
   (c) 60%
   (d) 70%
   (e) 90%

23. When should a periodontal assessment generally be repeated following non-surgical treatment?
   (a) Two weeks
   (b) One month
   (c) Three months
   (d) Six months
   (e) One year

24. Which of the following is not a risk factor for periodontal disease?
   (a) Smoking
   (b) Fizzy drinks
   (c) Diabetes
   (d) Plaque
   (e) Genetics

25. Which of the following is not a feature usually seen in necrotising ulcerative periodontitis (NUP)?
   (a) Ulcerated interdental papillae
   (b) Pain
   (c) Bleeding
   (d) Halitosis
   (e) Salty taste

21. c

Treponema denticola is a small, thin, gram-negative spirochaete.

22. d

Roughly 70% of plaque is formed of micro-organisms, with the remaining 30% being formed by the interbacterial matrix.

23. c

Periodontal assessment should be repeated three months following root surface debridement. This will allow assessment of success of treatment and whether further treatment is necessary.

24. b

Fizzy drinks are not associated with periodontal diseases. They would more commonly be linked with erosion and caries.

25. e

Generally, a metallic taste rather than a salty taste is reported in this condition. NUP can be quite a painful condition and requires antibiotic treatment.

26. Which antibiotic is usually prescribed for NUP?
  (a) Amoxicillin
  (b) Penicillin
  (c) Metronidazole
  (d) Clindamycin
  (e) Vancomycin

27. Which instrument is shown in the following photograph?

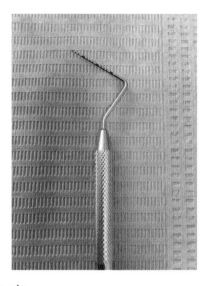

  (a) UNC-15 probe
  (b) Marquis probe
  (c) Williams probe
  (d) CPITN probe
  (e) Naber's probe

28. Based on the updated periodontal classification system, what stage would a patient with clinical attachment loss of 3–4 mm be classed as?
  (a) Stage V
  (b) Stage II
  (c) Stage I
  (d) Stage III
  (e) Stage IV

26. c

Typically, a three-day course of metronidazole is given to the patient (400 mg TDS). Along with this, a hydrogen peroxide mouthwash, local measures and oral hygiene instructions are given to the patient.

27. a

This is a UNC-15 probe which has incremental markings at every millimetre. There are then black bands between 4–5, 9–10 and 14–15 mm. The standard periodontal probe, used for assessment, is the CPITN probe.

28. b

The staging is broken down in the table below:

	Periodontitis	Stage I	Stage II	Stage III	Stage IV
Severity	Clinical attachment loss	1–2 mm	3–4 mm	≥5 mm	≥5 mm
	Radiographic bone loss	Coronal third (<15%)	Coronal (15–33%)	Middle or apical third of the root	Middle or apical third of the root
	Tooth loss due to periodontitis	No tooth loss		≤4 teeth	≥5 teeth
Complexity		Maximum probing depth ≤4 mm. Mostly horizontal bone loss	Maximum probing depth ≤5 mm. Mostly horizontal bone loss	In addition to Stage II: Probing depth ≥6 mm Vertical bone loss ≥3 mm Class II or III furcation involvement Moderate ridge defects	In addition to Stage III: Need for complex rehabilitation due to masticatory dysfunction, tooth mobility, bite collapse, pathological migration, or <20 remaining teeth
Extent and distribution		Localised (<30% of teeth involved) Generalised (≥30% of teeth involved) Molar-incisor pattern			

29. Which of the following would fall in Grade C criteria for periodontitis?
   (a) No bone loss over five years
   (b) <10 cigarettes a day
   (c) HbA1c≥7%
   (d) % bone loss/age of between 0.25 and 1
   (e) Non-smoker

30. A patient presents with pocket probing depths 5–6 mm throughout their mouth. Radiographs demonstrate bone loss of around 30%. Their % bone loss/age is 0.6. Based on this information, what would their diagnosis be using the updated periodontal classification system?
   (a) Generalised periodontitis; Stage II/Grade C
   (b) Localised periodontitis; Stage IV/Grade B
   (c) Generalised periodontitis; Stage II/Grade B
   (d) Generalised periodontitis; Stage III/Grade B
   (e) Localised periodontitis; Stage III/Grade B

29. c

The grading is broken down in the table below:

	Progression		Grade A: Slow rate	Grade B: Moderate rate	Grade C: Rapid rate
Primary criteria	Direct evidence of progression	Radiographic bone loss or clinical attachment level	No loss over five years	<2 mm over five years	≥2 mm over five years
	Indirect evidence of progression	% Bone loss/ age	<0.25	0.25–1.0	>1.0
		Case phenotype	Heavy biofilm with low levels of destruction	Destruction commensurate with biofilm deposits	Destruction inconsistent with biofilm deposits; clinical patterns suggestive of period of rapid progression and/or early onset
Grade modifiers	Risk factors	Smoking	Non-smoker	<10 cigarettes/ day	≥10 cigarettes/day
		Diabetes	Non-diabetic	Diabetic with HbA1c<7%	Diabetic with HbA1c≥7%

30. d

As the majority of their mouth demonstrates probing depths of 5–6 mm, this would constitute generalised periodontitis. Check the tables presented in Answers 28 and 29 for the full breakdown.

CHAPTER 7

Pharmacology and Human Disease

Single Best Answer Questions for Dentistry, First Edition. Prateek Biyani.
© 2021 John Wiley & Sons Ltd. Published 2021 by John Wiley & Sons Ltd.

1. Which of the following analgesics is the safest to prescribe to a pregnant woman?
   (a) Ibuprofen
   (b) Diclofenac
   (c) Paracetamol
   (d) Aspirin
   (e) Co-codamol

2. Which of the following is not a non-steroidal anti-inflammatory drug (NSAID)?
   (a) Ibuprofen
   (b) Codeine
   (c) Diclofenac
   (d) Aspirin
   (e) Ketoprofen

3. Which of the following drugs is a short-acting beta-agonist (SABA)?
   (a) Salbutamol
   (b) Salmeterol
   (c) Tiotropium bromide
   (d) Prednisolone
   (e) Formoterol

4. Anaphylactic reaction is which of the following?
   (a) Type IV hypersensitivity
   (b) Type I hypersensitivity
   (c) Type III hypersensitivity
   (d) Type II hypersensitivity
   (e) Type V hypersensitivity

5. A 56-year-old man reports suffering from a sudden shortness in breath with a sharp pain upon inhaling, without any stimulus. He has recently been in hospital for surgery and is a long-term warfarin user. What is the most likely cause of his symptoms?
   (a) Cardiac failure
   (b) Pulmonary embolism (PE)
   (c) Muscle pain
   (d) Choking
   (e) Asthma attack

1. c

Paracetamol is the safest analgesic that could be prescribed. NSAIDs should be avoided due to the multiple risks they pose to the mother and baby during pregnancy and afterwards. Aspirin is also associated with the development of Reye's syndrome.

2. b

Codeine is an opiate and has the same mechanism of action as morphine.

3. a

Salbutamol is the most common drug found in inhalers given in asthma and is usually the 'blue' inhaler. Salmeterol and formoterol are examples of long-acting beta-agonists. Tiotropium bromide is an example of a long-acting muscarinic antagonist and prednisolone is a steroid.

4. b

Anaphylaxis occurs as an acute type I hypersensitivity reaction.

5. b

This is most likely a PE given the symptoms and history of surgery and warfarin. As there is no obvious stimulus, it is unlikely to be an asthma attack.

6. Which of the following is not a symptom of tuberculosis (TB)?
   (a) Persistent cough
   (b) Weight loss
   (c) Fever
   (d) Night sweats
   (e) Increased appetite

7. Infective endocarditis can present with which of the following symptoms?
   (a) Swan neck fingers
   (b) Target lesions
   (c) Splinter haemorrhages
   (d) Arthritis
   (e) Nodules

8. Which of the following is an ACE inhibitor?
   (a) Losartan
   (b) Ramipril
   (c) Atenolol
   (d) Doxazosin
   (e) Amlodipine

9. What is the mechanism of action of beta-lactam antibiotics?
   (a) Inhibit bacterial cell wall synthesis
   (b) Inhibit ribosomal activity at the 30S site
   (c) Inhibit ribosomal activity at the 50S site
   (d) Inhibit DNA synthesis
   (e) Inhibit peptidoglycan cross-linkage

10. Which of the following is not a sign of chronic liver disease?
   (a) Jaundice
   (b) Finger clubbing
   (c) Spider naevi
   (d) Pale stools
   (e) Ascites

6. e

TB commonly causes patients to lose significant weight. It is commonly associated with fevers, night sweats, fatigue and a persistent, often productive, cough.

7. c

Splinter haemorrhages are a common presentation in infective endocarditis, caused by small clots in the nail beds.

8. b

Ramipril is an ACE inhibitor and works by preventing the conversion of angiotensin I to angiotensin II. Losartan is an angiotensin II receptor antagonist; atenolol is a beta-blocker; doxazosin is an alpha-blocker; and amlodipine is a calcium channel antagonist.

9. a

Beta-lactams, such as amoxicillin, work through inhibiting bacterial cell wall and peptidoglycan synthesis. Antibiotics that target the 30S ribosomal site include tetracyclines and aminoglycosides. Macrolides, such as erythromycin, target the 50S ribosomal site. Metronidazole works by targeting and disrupting DNA synthesis. Peptidoglycan cross-linkage is inhibited by vancomycin.

10. d

Dark stools are more commonly seen in chronic liver disease.

11. A 32-year-old man presents with a dental abscess, swelling and lymphadenopathy. Which of the following antibiotics would be most appropriate?
    (a) Gentamicin
    (b) Amoxicillin
    (c) Tetracycline
    (d) Erythromycin
    (e) Cefotaxime

12. Which of the following anaesthetics is associated with methaemaglobinaemia when given in large doses?
    (a) Procaine
    (b) Cocaine
    (c) Articaine
    (d) Lignocaine
    (e) Prilocaine

13. Why is adrenaline added to local anaesthetics?
    (a) It is a vehicle for the anaesthetic
    (b) It increases blood flow to the area
    (c) It increases the absorption of the anaesthetic
    (d) It decreases the patient's heart rate
    (e) It increases the duration of the anaesthetic

14. A 40-year-old patient complains of severe pain along the right side of her jaw and face. Which of the following is the best choice of drug to manage neuralgic pain?
    (a) Paracetamol
    (b) Carbamazepine
    (c) Ibuprofen
    (d) Metronidazole
    (e) Aciclovir

15. Which of the following would not usually be prescribed to someone suffering from gastro-oesophageal reflux disease (GORD)?
    (a) Omeprazole
    (b) Lansoprazole
    (c) Ranitidine
    (d) Ibuprofen
    (e) Cimetidine

11. b

Amoxicillin is generally the first-choice antibiotic for dental abscesses. Metronidazole is often an alternative. Erythromycin may sometimes be considered as a third-line option.

12. e

This is a rare complication associated with prilocaine and may present with shortness of breath, cyanosis and headaches.

13. e

Adrenaline causes vasoconstriction which allows the anaesthetic to remain in the operative area for longer.

14. b

Carbamazepine is one of the drugs of choice for neuralgic pain, along with other drugs such as gabapentin. The other medications would have limited benefit in this case.

15. d

Ibuprofen is likely to exacerbate the patient's GORD and increases the risk of gastric ulceration.

16. A 50-year-old patient presents with a medical history stating he suffers from renal disease. Which of the following symptoms is he unlikely to suffer from?
    (a) Hypotension
    (b) Anaemia
    (c) Lethargy
    (d) Pruritus
    (e) Loss of appetite

17. Which of the following is an acute complication of diabetes mellitus?
    (a) Retinopathy
    (b) Nephropathy
    (c) Ischaemic heart disease
    (d) Diabetic ketoacidosis
    (e) Neuropathy

18. A 34-year-old patient attends his recall appointment. He states that he recently had a bout of fever, nausea and vomiting. He has recently been on a trip to India. Which of the following could be the cause of this?
    (a) Hepatitis B
    (b) Hepatitis C
    (c) Cytomegalovirus
    (d) Hepatitis E
    (e) Human papillomavirus

19. A patient presents with pain from a lower right tooth. He suffers from rheumatoid arthritis. Which of the following is not associated with his condition?
    (a) Rheumatic nodules
    (b) Atlantoaxial subluxation
    (c) Stiff joints
    (d) Flexible skin
    (e) Swan neck fingers

20. What is the inheritance for Haemophilia A?
    (a) Autosomal dominant
    (b) Autosomal recessive
    (c) X-linked recessive
    (d) X-linked dominant
    (e) It is not inherited

16. a

Renal disease would cause hypertension due to the fluid retention.

17. d

All the others are chronic complications associated with diabetes mellitus.

18. d

Hepatitis E is commonly contracted in countries like India. It presents with nausea, fatigue and jaundice. It is generally an acute infection but can have chronic effects in immunocompromised patients.

19. d

Flexible skin is usually associated with collagen disorders such as Ehlers-Danlos syndrome.

20. c

Haemophilia A is a deficiency in factor XIII. It has X-linked recessive inheritance, causing the phenotype to be expressed in males whilst females are usually carriers.

21. Which of the following may present with neurosyphilis, aortic lesions and bone deformities?
    (a) Primary syphilis
    (b) Secondary syphilis
    (c) Latent syphilis
    (d) Tertiary syphilis
    (e) None of the above

22. Which of the following is administered in the event of paracetamol overdose?
    (a) Naloxone
    (b) N-acetylcysteine
    (c) Protamine sulphate
    (d) Water
    (e) Ibuprofen

23. Which of the following does not have a vaccine?
    (a) Meningitis C
    (b) Meningitis A
    (c) Meningitis B
    (d) Meningitis Y
    (e) Meningitis W135

24. Which of the following is not a known side effect associated with the use of prednisolone?
    (a) Weight gain
    (b) Hyperglycaemia
    (c) Increased infection
    (d) Reduced appetite
    (e) Nausea

25. Which of the following is a medication commonly prescribed to patients suffering from atrial fibrillation?
    (a) Ibuprofen
    (b) Digoxin
    (c) Carbamazepine
    (d) Methotrexate
    (e) Heparin

21. d

These are symptoms associated with tertiary syphilis, an infection caused by the bacteria *Treponema pallidum*. Tertiary syphilis is rarely seen in the developed world.

22. b

N-acetylcysteine is used as treatment. Naloxone is used in the event of opiate overdose and protamine sulphate is used with heparin.

23. c

Meningitis B currently does not have a vaccine as it is too variable. The other strains do have vaccines available.

24. d

Steroids tend to increase appetite and, hence, weight gain.

25. b

Digoxin is commonly prescribed for atrial fibrillation, atrial flutter and sometimes heart failure.

26. Barrett's oesophagus describes which of the following?
  (a) Swelling in the upper portion of the oesophagus
  (b) Change in epithelium type along the lining of the oesophagus
  (c) A developmental abnormality causing narrowing of the oesophagus
  (d) A shortening of the oesophagus
  (e) Abnormal polyps along the oesophagus

27. Addison's disease is characterised as which of the following?
  (a) Hypothyroidism
  (b) Hyperthyroidism
  (c) Hypocortisolism
  (d) Hypercortisolism
  (e) Hypopituitarism

28. Which of the following cranial nerves provides motor supply to the tongue?
  (a) CN IV
  (b) CN V
  (c) CN VII
  (d) CN X
  (e) CN XII

29. Which of the following is not a side effect of codeine phosphate?
  (a) Drowsiness
  (b) Diarrhoea
  (c) Nausea
  (d) Anaphylaxis
  (e) Respiratory depression

30. What is the usual oral dose of metronidazole prescribed to patients?
  (a) 200 mg TDS
  (b) 200 mg BD
  (c) 400 mg BD
  (d) 400 mg TDS
  (e) 500 mg TDS

26. b

This is considered to be a premalignant condition and is caused by metaplastic changes occurring towards the lower portion of the oesophagus.

27. c

Addison's disease occurs due to a lack of cortisol and is an autoimmune condition. It presents with weakness, hypotension, hypoglycaemia and loss of weight. Increased cortisol levels cause Cushing's syndrome.

28. e

Cranial nerve XII is the hypoglossal nerve and supplies motor innervation to the tongue. Damage to it will cause deviation of the tongue.

29. b

Codeine phosphate typically causes constipation as opposed to diarrhoea.

30. d

Metronidazole is typically prescribed at a dose of 400 mg TDS orally. When given IV, it is prescribed as 500 mg TDS.

CHAPTER 8
Dental Materials

Single Best Answer Questions for Dentistry, First Edition. Prateek Biyani.
© 2021 John Wiley & Sons Ltd. Published 2021 by John Wiley & Sons Ltd.

1. Which of the following defines a metal?
   (a) A crystalline structure held together by ionic bonds
   (b) An amorphous structure held together by ionic bonds
   (c) A crystalline structure held together by metallic bonds
   (d) A long chain molecule held together by covalent bonds
   (e) An amorphous structure held together by metallic bonds

2. How many clinical stages are required for dentine bonding agents?
   (a) Dentine bonding agents are not required
   (b) One step
   (c) Two steps
   (d) Three steps
   (e) Depends on the agent

3. Which of the following chemicals is commonly used as an initiator in polymerisation reactions?
   (a) Benzoyl peroxide
   (b) Water
   (c) Sodium chloride
   (d) Calcium bicarbonate
   (e) Fluoroaluminosilicate glass

4. Which of the following is not a component of calcium hydroxide liners?
   (a) Calcium hydroxide
   (b) Zinc oxide
   (c) Zinc stearate
   (d) Fillers
   (e) Ethanol

5. Which of the following is the main component of alginate?
   (a) Calcium alginate
   (b) Sodium phosphate
   (c) Sodium alginate
   (d) Water
   (e) Potassium sulphate

1. c

a and **b** describe ceramics, whilst **d** best describes a polymer.

2. e

The number of stages depends on the agent used, varying from one to three steps. For example, some agents may have combined etching and bonding properties, reducing the clinical stages.

3. a

An initiator triggers the polymerisation reaction to begin. Usually some form of activation is required to start the process and this may be in the form of light or heat.

4. e

Ethanol is not found in this liner.

5. c

Sodium alginate is the main component of alginate. Sodium phosphate and potassium sulphate are also required, but in lesser quantities.

6. Which of the following best describes amalgam?
   (a) Substitutional solid solution
   (b) Intermetallic compound
   (c) Interstitial solid solution
   (d) Pure metal
   (e) Amorphous ceramic

7. Which of these is not a property of alginate?
   (a) Relatively cheap
   (b) Easy to manipulate
   (c) Dimensionally stable
   (d) Low tear strength
   (e) Rapid set

8. Which of the following is not an elastic impression material?
   (a) Agar
   (b) Alginate
   (c) Polyether
   (d) Addition cured silicone
   (e) Impression compound

9. Which of the following is not an advantage of adhesive materials?
   (a) Conservation of tooth structure
   (b) Reduction in marginal leakage
   (c) Reinforcement of weakened tooth structure
   (d) Reduced cost
   (e) Reduced postoperative sensitivity

10. Calcium hydroxide does not have which of the following properties?
    (a) Easy to mix
    (b) Adhesive
    (c) Highly soluble
    (d) Highly alkaline
    (e) Low strength

6. b

Amalgam is a type of metal alloy which has metals mixed at a particular stoichiometric ratio.

7. c

Alginate is a commonly used primary impression material, but it suffers from poor dimensional stability. This is because, if left in improper conditions, it can be affected by imbibition or syneresis.

8. e

Impression compound is a rigid impression material, more suited for edentulous patients.

9. d

Generally, adhesive materials have a higher cost than alternatives.

10. b

Calcium hydroxide is non-adhesive, but due to its high pH it is thought to be antibacterial.

11. What percentage of phosphoric acid is commonly used to etch enamel?
    (a) 1%
    (b) 5%
    (c) 35%
    (d) 75%
    (e) 100%

12. How does etching enamel improve adhesion?
    (a) Creates a micromechanically retentive surface
    (b) Increases surface area for bonding
    (c) Reduces surface energy to improve wettability
    (d) a and b
    (e) a, b and c

13. What are the three basic steps, in the correct order, in any dentine bonding agent?
    (a) Etch, seal, cure
    (b) Etch, prime, seal
    (c) Prime, etch, cure
    (d) Prime, etch, seal
    (e) Etch, dry, seal

14. Which of the following describes the gamma-1 phase in an amalgam reaction?
    (a) Hg
    (b) Ag_2Hg_3
    (c) Ag_3Sn
    (d) Ag_3Sn_3
    (e) Sn_7Hg

15. Which of the following is the problematic component of amalgam?
    (a) Hg
    (b) Ag_2Hg_3
    (c) Ag_3Sn
    (d) Ag_3Sn_3
    (e) Sn_7Hg

11. c

35% phosphoric acid is commonly used to etch enamel and dentine prior to restoring.

12. d

Etching enamel raises the surface energy and thus improves wettability.

13. b

Dentine bonding agents require etching, priming and finally sealing for correct bonding. These can be done in various combinations but must be in this order.

14. b

c describes the gamma phase of the reaction whilst e describes the gamma-2 phase.

15. e

The gamma-2 phase is responsible for corrosion as well as reducing the overall strength of the amalgam. This is reduced by dispersed-phase amalgams containing copper.

16. Which of the following is not an action of fillers in composite?
    (a) Reduce polymerisation shrinkage
    (b) Provide radiopacity
    (c) Increase coefficient of thermal expansion
    (d) Control aesthetic properties
    (e) Increase wear resistance

17. What is the average size of filler particles in microfilled resins?
    (a) 1 μm
    (b) 0.5 μm
    (c) 0.05 μm
    (d) 0.005 μm
    (e) 0.001 μm

18. Which of the following describes the release of calcium ions in the setting of GIC?
    (a) Hardening
    (b) Gelation
    (c) Chelation
    (d) Dissolution
    (e) Precipitation

19. Which is the softest type of gold alloy?
    (a) Type II
    (b) Type I
    (c) Type IV
    (d) Type IIII
    (e) Type V

20. Which of the following is not an advantage of zinc phosphate cements?
    (a) Low cost
    (b) Easy to use
    (c) Long working time
    (d) Short setting time
    (e) Adequate compressive strength

16. c

Fillers reduce the coefficient of thermal expansion, with the aim to bring it as close to enamel and dentine to reduce stress.

17. c

This is the average size of filler particles in microfilled resins.

18. b

Gelation describes the process of release of calcium ions and subsequent cross-linking in the material.

19. b

Type I is the softest alloy and type IV is the hardest. Type III gold is most commonly used in dentistry.

20. d

Zinc phosphate cement has a long setting time and thus this is a disadvantage clinically.

21. Which of the following is tartaric acid responsible for in GIC?
  (a) Improving aesthetics
  (b) Allowing bulk fill
  (c) Even dispensing
  (d) Controls working and setting times
  (e) Increases strength

22. Which of the following is an inhibitor often used in denture acrylic?
  (a) Methyl methacrylate
  (b) Benzoyl peroxide
  (c) Hydroquinone
  (d) Ethylene glycol dimethacrylate
  (e) Ethyl acrylate

23. Which of the following is the cross-linking agent in denture acrylic?
  (a) Methyl methacrylate
  (b) Benzoyl peroxide
  (c) Hydroquinone
  (d) Ethylene glycol dimethacrylate
  (e) Ethyl acrylate

24. What percentage of gold is found in type III high-gold alloys?
  (a) 50%
  (b) 60%
  (c) 70%
  (d) 85%
  (e) 90%

25. Which of the following best describes the term 'stiffness'?
  (a) The ability of a material to resist crack propagation
  (b) The maximum amount of energy a material can absorb
  (c) The ability of a structure to maintain its shape when acted upon by a load
  (d) The process of crack propagation under cyclic loads
  (e) The displacement of material at the surface

21. d

Tartaric acid helps control working and setting times by isolating calcium ions and preventing cross-linking.

22. c

Hydroquinone is the inhibitor which helps increase the shelf-life of the material.

23. d

Ethylene glycol dimethacrylate helps to cross-link the polymers and improve the physical properties of the material.

24. c

Type III high-gold alloys usually contain between 62% and 78% gold.

25. c

Stiffness is the ability of a structure to maintain its shape when acted upon by a load. Toughness refers to the resistance to crack propagation.

26. What are the three main components of composite resins?
(a) Resin matrix, filler, coupling agent
(b) Resin matrix, coupling agent, etch
(c) Resin matrix, filler, etch
(d) Resin matrix, bond, coupling agent
(e) Resin matrix, adhesive, filler

27. What is the wavelength of light typically used to cure composite resins?
(a) 200 nm
(b) 340 nm
(c) 380 nm
(d) 470 nm
(e) 500 nm

28. What is generally the maximum accepted thickness of composite resin that can be effectively cured by a light?
(a) 1 mm
(b) 1.5 mm
(c) 2 mm
(d) 2.5 mm
(e) 3 mm

26. a

Composite resins are made of three components including the resin matrix, filler and coupling agent. Composite resins then require etching and bonding to the tooth surface.

27. d

A blue light of wavelength between 470 and 480 nm is usually used to cure composite resins. There are various types of lights that exist, including halogen and LED.

28. c

Generally, 2 mm is accepted as the maximum thickness of composite that should be cured at a time. This therefore dictates the increments of composite that should be used.

CHAPTER 9
Radiology

Study the OPT below and answer the following questions.

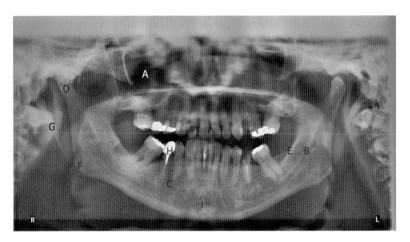

1. Which of the labels represents the mental foramen?
   (a) A
   (b) B
   (c) C
   (d) F
   (e) I

2. Which space is identified by A?
   (a) Frontal sinus
   (b) Ethmoid sinus
   (c) Nasal cavity
   (d) Maxillary sinus
   (e) Oropharynx

3. What is supplied by the structure passing through B?
   (a) Motor function to lower lip
   (b) Sensation to upper lip
   (c) Sensation to lower lip
   (d) Motor function to tongue
   (e) Sensation to maxillary teeth

1. c

This is the mental foramen where the mental nerve, a branch of the inferior alveolar nerve, exits.

2. d

A identifies the maxillary sinus – the frontal and ethmoid sinuses cannot normally be seen on an OPT.

3. c

The structure passing through **B** is the inferior alveolar nerve which supplies sensation to the lower lip, as well as the mandibular teeth, some of the buccal mucosa and the chin.

4. Which of the following labels the external oblique ridge?

(a) G
(b) F
(c) I
(d) E
(e) D

5. The image below shows a holder for which type of radiograph?

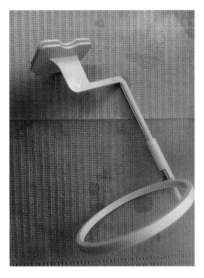

(a) Anterior periapical
(b) Bitewing
(c) Posterior periapical
(d) Endodontic periapical
(e) Upper standard occlusal

4. d

This is the external oblique ridge which is a common landmark for procedures including delivering inferior alveolar nerve blocks as well as surgical extraction of wisdom teeth.

5. b

This is the typical holder for a bitewing radiograph, primarily used to detect caries.

Study the OPT below and answer the following questions.

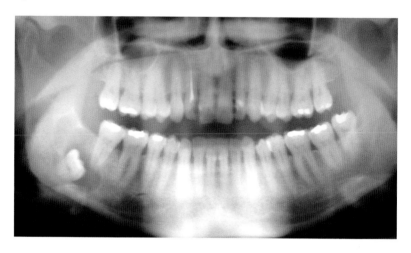

6. Which tooth has been root treated?
   (a) UL2
   (b) UR2
   (c) UL1
   (d) UL3
   (e) UR3

7. How would you describe the main lesion identified on this radiograph?
   (a) Well-defined radiopacity
   (b) Ill-defined radiolucency
   (c) Ill-defined radiopacity
   (d) Well-defined radiolucency
   (e) Mixed radiodensity

8. Which of the following is the most likely diagnosis for the lesion identified?
   (a) Squamous cell carcinoma
   (b) Ameloblastoma
   (c) Odontogenic keratocyst
   (d) Dentigerous cyst
   (e) Odontome

6. b

The UR2, or upper right 2, has been root treated which is evident by the radiopaque root canal.

7. d

The lesion surrounding the LR8 is a well-defined radiolucency.

8. d

This is due to the well-defined radiolucency being attached at the ACJ of the LR8. Other differentials, but less likely, are ameloblastoma and odontogenic keratocyst. An odontome would generally be mixed density or radiopaque, whilst a squamous cell carcinoma would be poorly defined.

9. What would be a potential concern during removal of this lesion?
   (a) Loss of motor innervation to the cheek
   (b) Loss of sensation to the upper lip
   (c) Loss of motor innervation to the lower lip
   (d) Loss of sensation to the lower lip
   (e) Loss of motor innervation to the chin

10. Which combination of radiographs should be taken to assess a mandibular fracture?
   (a) Bitewing and periapical
   (b) Upper standard occlusal and OPT
   (c) OPT and PA mandible
   (d) PA mandible and lateral cephalogram
   (e) CT and PA mandible

11. Which of the following conditions is associated with multiple odontogenic keratocysts?
   (a) Apert's syndrome
   (b) Down's syndrome
   (c) Gardner's syndrome
   (d) Gorlin–Goltz syndrome
   (e) Burning mouth syndrome

12. Which radiographic views would be requested for a fractured zygoma?
   (a) OPT and PA mandible
   (b) OPT and OM 0°
   (c) OM 0° and OM 30°
   (d) OM 30° and upper standard occlusion
   (e) OPT and OM 30°

9. d

There would be a risk of damage to the inferior alveolar nerve and, therefore, sensation to the lower lip.

10. c

This is the usual first-line combination and helps to assess displacement in every axis. A CT scan may be required at a later date to assess further damage.

11. d

Gorlin–Goltz syndrome is associated with multiple odontogenic keratocysts, as well as basal cell carcinomas. Gardner's syndrome leads to multiple jaw osteomas as well as intestinal polyps.

12. c

This is the best combination to assess a fractured zygoma, allowing the clinician to see the bones from two different views and assess for displacement.

Study the OPT below and answer the following questions.

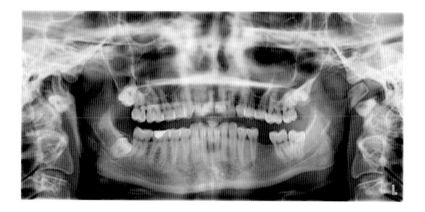

13. Which of the teeth is most likely to be prevented from eruption?
    (a) LL8
    (b) UL8
    (c) UR8
    (d) LR8
    (e) None

14. Which of the following faults has most likely occurred in this radiograph?
    (a) Patient has moved
    (b) Patient is too far out of the machine
    (c) Patient is too far into the machine
    (d) Patient has their chin up
    (e) Patient has their chin down

15. Which of the following best describes a Stafne defect?
    (a) Ill-defined radiolucency below the inferior dental canal
    (b) Well-defined radiolucency above the inferior dental canal
    (c) Ill-defined radiolucency above the inferior dental canal
    (d) Well-defined radiolucency below the inferior dental canal
    (e) Well-defined radiolucency above the mental foramen

13. b

There appears to be an obstruction associated with the UL8 crown – this could be a supernumerary tooth or an odontome.

14. c

The patient appears to be too far into the machine, hence the spine is in complete view. If the patient was in chin up or down then this would move the occlusal table.

15. d

Stafne defects are thought to be caused by excess salivary gland tissue. They are well-defined, unilocular radiolucencies found below the inferior dental canal.

16. A well-defined radiopaque lesion associated with the root of a lower right first molar is most likely to be a/an:
    (a) Periapical abscess
    (b) Cementoblastoma
    (c) Odontogenic keratocyst
    (d) Ameloblastoma
    (e) Osteoma

17. According to the Ionising Radiations Regulations 2017 (IRR17), what is the dose limit to the general public?
    (a) 0.5 mSv
    (b) 1 mSv
    (c) 2 mSv
    (d) 5 mSv
    (e) 10 mSv

18. What is the radiation exposure from a bitewing radiograph?
    (a) 0.0005 mSv
    (b) 0.0001 mSv
    (c) 0.05 mSv
    (d) 0.01 mSv
    (e) 0.005 mSv

19. Which of the following would not be seen in dentinogenesis imperfecta?
    (a) Short roots
    (b) Large pulp chambers
    (c) Lack of enamel
    (d) Bulbous crowns
    (e) Slender roots

20. Which radiograph would be most suitable for submandibular salivary stones?
    (a) OPT
    (b) PA mandible
    (c) Lower standard occlusal
    (d) Bitewing
    (e) Lateral cephalogram

16. b

As this is associated with the root of the tooth, it is most likely a cementoblastoma. These are well defined and usually radiopaque, often with a radiolucent rim.

17. b

1 mSv is the limit for the general public. The limit for classified workers is 20 and 6 mSv for non-classified workers.

18. e

Bitewing radiographs tend to cause 0.005 mSv of radiation exposure, whilst OPTs are responsible for 0.01 mSv.

19. b

The pulp chambers tend to be absent along with the root canals, therefore it is unusual to see large pulp chambers.

20. c

A lower standard occlusal will best demonstrate the position and size of a submandibular stone. An OPT can sometimes be the first point of detection.

21. Which of the following is not a method of reducing radiation exposure?
   (a) Collimation
   (b) Filtration
   (c) High kilovoltage
   (d) Fastest possible film
   (e) Lead shielding

22. Which of the following refers to 'effects that occur by chance when exposed with radiation'?
   (a) Deterministic effects
   (b) Stochastic effects
   (c) Non-stochastic effects
   (d) Therapeutic effects
   (e) Contactable effects

23. Who is responsible for justifying the radiation exposure during a dental radiograph?
   (a) The referrer
   (b) The practitioner
   (c) The operator
   (d) The patient
   (e) None of the above

24. Which of the following is not an indication for a periapical radiograph?
   (a) Assessment of root morphology
   (b) Assessment of periodontal status
   (c) Assessment of apical infection
   (d) Endodontic assessment
   (e) Assessment of caries

25. Which of the following is not an acceptable localisation technique for ectopic canines?
   (a) Vertical parallax – OPT and upper standard occlusal
   (b) Cone-beam CT
   (c) Horizontal parallax – two periapical radiographs
   (d) Horizontal parallax – upper standard occlusal and bitewing radiograph
   (e) Conventional CT

21. c

A kilovoltage of between 60 and 70 kVp should typically be used. Anything above this does not add any diagnostic value but increases the dosage. Filtration is crucial to removing low-energy photons from the beam, which would otherwise just be absorbed by the skin.

22. b

Stochastic effects refer to effects that occur by chance when exposed to radiation. Deterministic effects are dose dependent.

23. b

The referrer is responsible for providing enough clinical evidence to justify the radiograph. The practitioner is responsible for justifying the exposure. The operator is responsible for carrying out the radiation exposure.

24. e

Bitewing radiographs are the gold standard for caries diagnosis.

25. d

An upper standard occlusal and a bitewing radiograph would not constitute parallax in the horizontal plane.

26. Which nerve is most commonly damaged during a zygomatic arch fracture?
   (a) CN VII
   (b) CN VI
   (c) CN V
   (d) CN IV
   (e) CN III

27. Which of the following would present as a well-defined, unilocular radiolucency at the apex of a tooth, consistent with the lamina dura?
   (a) Dentigerous cyst
   (b) Eruption cyst
   (c) Osteoma
   (d) Cementoblastoma
   (e) Radicular cyst

26. c

The fifth cranial nerve is the trigeminal nerve. This supplies the sensation to the majority of the face. During a zygomatic fracture, the maxillary division, particularly the infraorbital nerve, is commonly damaged.

27. e

Radicular cysts are signs of chronic apical infection in a tooth. Osteomas and cementoblastomas appear as radiopaque lesions, but may be present at the apex. Eruption and dentigerous cysts would typically present around the crown of a tooth.

Index

Single Best Answer Questions for Dentistry, First Edition. Prateek Biyani.
© 2021 John Wiley & Sons Ltd. Published 2021 by John Wiley & Sons Ltd.